SPECIAL REPORT:

A DOCTOR'S PROVEN NEW WAY TO CONQUER BACK PAIN

by

John E. Eichenlaub, M. D.

PARKER PUBLISHING COMPANY
West Nyack, New York 10995

10 9 8 7 6 5 4 3 2 1

Library of Congress Cataloging-in-Publication Data

Eichenlaub, John E.
Special report : a doctor's proven new way to conquer back pain / by John E. Eichenlaub.

p. cm.
ISBN 0-13-827049-X
1. Backache—Popular works. I. Title.
RD771.B217E43 1991
617.5'64—dc20 92-28322
CIP

ISBN 0-13-827049-X

9 780138 270490 52495>

Parker Publishing Company
Professional Publishing
West Nyack, NY 10995
Simon & Schuster, A Paramount Communications Company

Printed in the United States of America

TABLE OF CONTENTS

WHAT THIS SPECIAL REPORT CAN DO FOR YOU

As a family physician, I've treated hundreds of backache patients without surgery. Heat and cold, strapping and massage, rest and exercise, and other noninvasive methods have cured almost all of them. And I've used a lot of these methods on myself. With the aid of the techniques detailed in this report I'm able to play golf or tennis almost every day.

In this easy-to-use guide, you'll find forty-seven specific measures that will help you eliminate back pain. These measures, which can all be carried out in your own home, apply to the following six common problems:

> The work-weary or overstressed back. No matter what the nature of the strain might be, the same home techniques will give relief because the enemy is always lactic acid. Overuse makes this irritant accumulate in your back muscles, which causes steady, aggravating pain.

> Back pain from nervous tension. Tight muscles work just as hard as working ones, and get just as sore. You'll find effective measures both for relief and for prevention of these miseries.

The strained, sprained, or twisted back. The measures you need to use here differ greatly from those advised above. In fact, what works best may be exactly the opposite of what you would use for muscular backache: cold rather than heat, for instance, and gentle rather than firm massage.

The arthritic back. Every one of your vertebrae shares two joints with each of its neighbors. That's more joints than you have in both hands and arms! No wonder arthritis sometimes strikes in your back. But you'll find six very effective remedies in this report.

The osteoporotic back. The "bowed back" of age doesn't get there overnight. I've had patients in their forties who suffered collapsed vertebrae with weeks of pain. Osteoporosis thins and weakens your bones, including vertebrae, which then crunch into themselves from body weight. I've explained in this report exactly how to get back on your feet after such an episode. Also, I've explained how you can tell ahead of time if you're prone to this condition, and how to prevent future problems.

Pain from a pinched nerve in your back. Some doctors recommend surgery if they even suspect a "ruptured disc." But resting in the jackknife position and the disc-retracting dangle often stave off the surgeons for good.

You'll also find a section devoted to preventing back strains and injuries, both at home and at work.

The home measures I've described help almost everyone who suffers from back pain. But you might still need or benefit from further help. You might need remedies which can't be bought without a prescription, or maneuvers which require special equipment. You might even need an injection or operation. As a family doctor, that's always been part of my job, too—to help patients get care from others which I can't give them myself. So I've included something on that subject: my last section tells you when you might get further help from a health professional—a physical therapist, vocational counselor, or other expert, as well as a family doctor or specialist.

You wouldn't have picked up this report unless you (or one of your loved ones) had some sort of back trouble. But please don't just flip to the section which covers that particular condition. One kind of back trouble often makes you more prone to others (as I know all too well with my own four varieties). Backstrain causes muscle spasm, which puts extra burdens on some spine joints. Any painful back condition limits your activities and makes osteoporosis more likely.

So read the whole book. Its specific home measures have helped me, they've helped my patients, and I'm sure that they can help you.

John E. Eichenlaub, M.D.

SECTION ONE

HOW TO RELIEVE OVERWORKED-MUSCLE PAIN

Every adult in the world has probably suffered from the pain of overworked muscles. You often get it when you do physical work, whether it's lifting a shovel or hefting a basket of wet clothes. You can get it when you move furniture around or lug home the results of a successful shopping trip.

You don't usually go to a doctor about this kind of pain; you've come to expect it. But that's no reason to keep suffering, when you can get quick relief with the methods in this section. You won't find them in any medical textbooks. I stumbled on the key element almost accidentally. Here's how it happened:

Whenever I drive an automobile for more than an hour or so, the back muscles at the base of my neck ache like a bad tooth. Rolling my head around makes the muscles snap, crackle, and pop, but it doesn't do much for the pain. Finally, one day I got so frustrated and angry that I just punched my fingertips into the muscles and gave them a rough massage. The aching pain vanished like magic!

So I asked myself what made my neck hurt in the first place.

Unaccustomed muscle use seemed the likely answer. I put one hand against my chin while driving along, and realized that my head bounced around constantly from road irregularities. I was using the very muscles which got sore to balance my head and counteract every bump and sway, dozens of times a minute.

Why did very firm massage give relief?

Every time a muscle contracts, it makes lactic acid, an irritant. When a muscle contracts very often or very intensely, it makes a lot of lactic acid. Unless your system carries away all the lactic acid promptly, it irritates your tissues.

My heavy massage milked out the acids through the lymph vessels. This firm massage will help you with most overworked muscle pain. Let's get specific:

DRIVER'S NECKBASE PAIN

What you feel:

Steady, increasing ache in muscles at the base of your neck.

Cause:

Accumulated lactic acid in muscles used to balance your head while driving over bumps and curves.

Ordinarily that lactic acid moves out of your tissue by way of lymph passages. Juices flow slowly in these tiny, thin-walled vessels. But you can speed that flow, move waste products out of the overwrought muscle, and restore comfort. Here's the technique:

Solution 1

1. Press the tip of one finger very firmly into the painful muscle.
2. While maintaining pressure, move your finger in circles as far as the elasticity of your skin readily permits for about 5 seconds.
3. Release the pressure. Move your finger to an adjacent portion of the sore muscle and move as above.
4. Continue until the pain goes away, showing that you have kneaded the acids out of all sore areas.

Shortly after I discovered this technique, I played golf with Harry P., who was playing very poorly. Afterward he explained that he hadn't been able to keep his mind on the game, trying to decide whether to go to his niece's wedding. He really wanted to go, but he hated to think of the driver's neckbase pain he would suffer on the long, bumpy drive.

I explained the lactic acid problem to Harry and taught him to knead the sore muscles, as I've described in Solution 1. Three weeks later, when we played golf again, Harry told me how much he had enjoyed the wedding. Driving 300 miles each way, mostly on poor roads, hadn't bothered him at all. By milking the lactic acid out of the muscles often, he had made the whole trip in perfect comfort.

Harry and I talked further, and decided that the only trouble with this method was duration of relief. The pain vanished instantly with deep, kneading massage, but it came back every 10 or 15 minutes. Between us, we worked out this way to prolong relief (or keep the misery from happening):

Solution 2

> Adjust your driving position so that your head rests against the "whiplash prevention support" which the manufacturer has placed just behind the area where your head normally rests. This braces your head to relieve part of the strain.

Some of my patients can't find a comfortable position that gives them head support. If that's your situation, you should try Solution 3.

Solution 3

1. Buy a small, firm rubber pillow and a 2- to 3-inch Velcro® patch.

2. Sew the prickly piece of Velcro® to the back of the pillow.

3. Adjust your driver's seat to a comfortable position, and place the pillow where you can rest your head snugly against it.

4. Sew the smooth piece of Velcro® to the seat back or head support to hold the pillow in position.

I've put driver's neckbase pain first in this report because it shows how rapidly very firm kneading of tired, aching muscles gives relief. This very heavy massage will help you whenever you suffer from fatigue-spurred muscle ache. As you now know, this most effective relief-giving measure moves accumulated acids into and through lymph vessels. Those vessels act like sponges: squeeze the liquid out and they'll soak up more irritating acid instantly! But it takes considerable pressure to empty them. And the <u>heavier</u> and the <u>tenser</u> the muscle, the more firmly you must knead.

Let's move on to another problem you're likely to have regularly:

HEAVY MUSCLE USE

<u>What you feel</u>:

Steady, dull back pain from your waist down to your hips.

<u>Cause</u>:

Enough muscle use to form more lactic acid than your system can carry away.

Shortly after I discovered how to get instant relief from driver's neckbase pain with heavy, kneading massage, Juan R. came to my office. As a migrant field worker, Juan spent all day bending and stooping. By quitting time, he could hardly straighten up. He spent each evening fighting the pain, mostly with tequila. A miserable life—bad enough that he thought seriously of throwing in the towel and going back to Mexico.

I started to shrug. No injury, no disease, just the

aftermaths of heavy work. Maybe he just couldn't hack that line of work.

Then I thought about the driver's neckbase misery we've just discussed. I explained to Juan how lactic acid piles up in a muscle when you use it over and over. And how he could move it out with very firm kneading.

Juan said that his wife would help. But she turned out to be so small and light that she couldn't press hard enough to milk acids out of the heavy muscles of Juan's back, especially when they were stiff and tight from pain. So the three of us worked out a way she could "roll away his pain." Here's the technique:

Solution 4

1. You can literally "roll away the pain" of a work-weary, aching back. For this method, you will need a willing helper, a 2-foot length of 1-inch × 10-inch smoothly finished wood, adhesive tape, and a tennis ball.
2. Wrap two or three thicknesses of tape around the board near each of its ends. Your helper will be holding on and pushing down on those areas, so they need to be smooth and slightly cushioned.
3. Lie on your stomach on a firm surface. (The floor works better than a soft bed.)

4. Have your helper kneel if necessary to let him or her carry out this technique comfortably.

5. Get him or her to put the tennis ball underneath the center of the board and against the middle of your worst aching muscle.

6. Get your helper to lean against both ends of the board, putting pressure on the tissue beneath the tennis ball.

7. Get your helper to move the board so that it rolls the ball along and across the aching muscle (Figure 1), moving acids into the lymph vessel "sponge".

8. As the pain disappears from each area, ask your helper to move up, down, or across

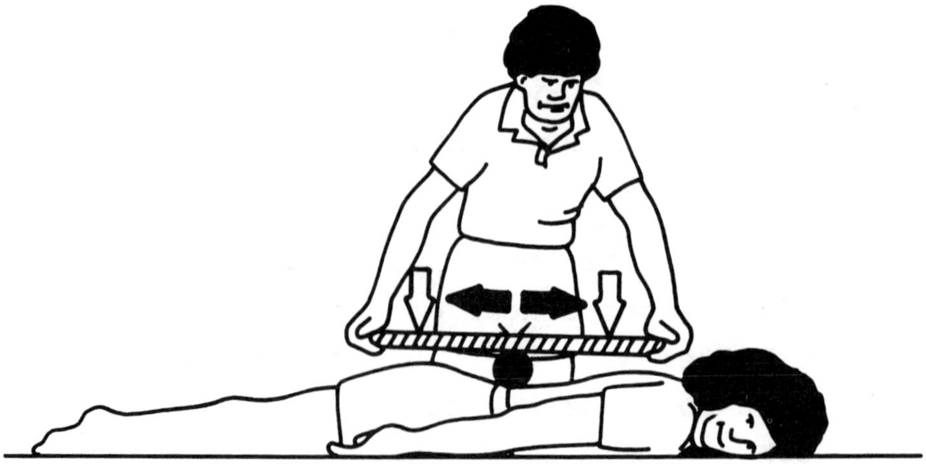

Figure 1

until all the ache-generating irritants have been milked out.

This technique works very well if your helper can exert (and you can tolerate) enough pressure to milk out the accumulated acids. But particularly if you're overweight, the tennis ball may give sufficiently intense pressure to be uncomfortable. If that happens, use this modification:

Solution 5

1. Get a larger ball, such as a seamless softball. Your helper will have to lean a little harder to make the less concentrated pressure suffice.

2. If this still causes discomfort, use a softer ball, like a children's rubber ball the same size as a softball. This spreads the pressure area even more and covers the area faster, but your helper will need to push very hard to milk out the acids.

When you find the degree of pressure which milks away the pain without causing too much discomfort, get your helper to "roll away the misery" from the entire aching area. You'll find that it gives incredible relief!

Here's a modification of the above technique to use when you don't have a helper:

Solution 6

1. Pick a smooth, solid wall which can't be damaged by a tennis ball, even when you're leaning hard against it.

2. If you don't have a suitable wall handy, buy a piece of Masonite for reinforcement.

3. Stand with your feet about 12 inches apart and with your heels about 18 inches from the wall.

4. Put a tennis ball between the wall and the center of one of your sore back muscles.

5. Lean solidly against the ball.

6. Bend your knees and roll your shoulders to move the ball across and along the sore muscle, always maintaining heavy pressure. (Figure 2) You will probably have to arch your back to bring the involved muscles into contact with the ball.

7. When you have "rolled the misery" out of one side of your back, put the ball near the center of the aching area on the other side of your spine and repeat the process.

8. Try a larger or softer ball after you have experienced the relief which a tennis ball can give. By leaning harder (since the pressure is spread over a larger area), you may be able to get similar relief more quickly.

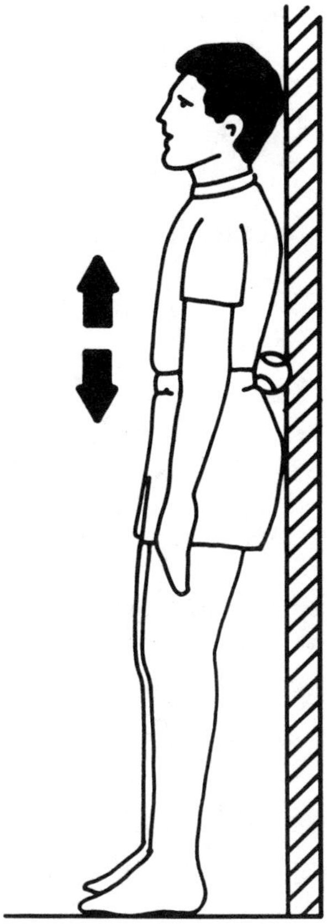

Figure 2

As I told you, what got me started on the "roll the pain away" technique was the slightness of Juan R.'s wife. She just didn't have the strength to milk acids out of Juan's sturdy back muscles with her fingertips.

Sven S.'s wife Solveig couldn't have been more different. A Nordic powerhouse, she practically dragged him to my office, complaining that he had turned into a "couch potato" who wouldn't take her anyplace or do anything with her. Sven explained that his job repairing track at the railroad left him with such a sore back that he just flopped in front of the TV most evenings and weekends. And his foreman had already warned him twice about slacking off.

Solveig obviously felt angry and rejected. But when I suggested that perhaps the whole problem could be solved with a variety of "Swedish" massage, she seemed willing to try. So the three of us worked out this next technique:

Solution 7

1. Lie on a firm surface, where your helper can comfortably reach (and press firmly on) your back.
2. Get your helper to spread some mineral oil over the area.
3. Get your helper to close both hands into fists and use the flat surfaces of the second finger segments (Figure 3) to press firmly into your aching muscles near the base of your spine and then (maintaining the pressure) slide both fists up along your back muscles to the rib cage.
4. Get him or her to repeat this action ten or twelve times, varying the site slightly to cover the entire width of the lengthwise back muscles.

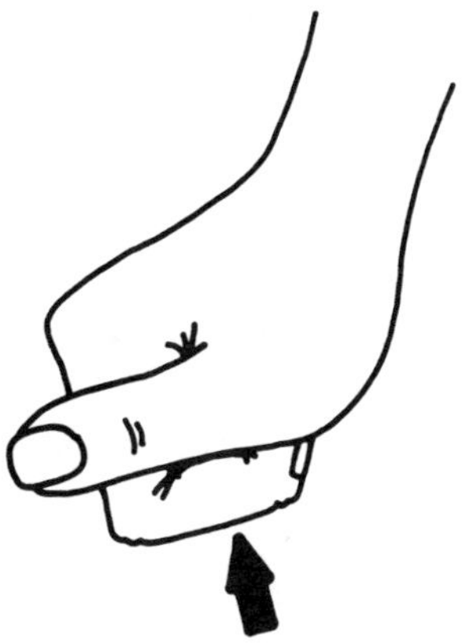

Figure 3

5. Your helper should then open his or her fists and stroke with firm fingertips diagonally from the center of your lower back toward both sides of your rib cage.

6. Finally, he or she should wipe off the oil with rubbing alcohol, which leaves you feeling clean and refreshed.

Sven and his wife worked this system into their daily routine, and it gave Sven new life. The massage instantly relieved his back pain, and his appreciation of Solveig's help with his problem made him more considerate. They started going places and doing things as a couple, and really enjoying each other. And, knowing he wouldn't have to suffer all evening, he started really extending himself at work. After about a year, the company made him foreman. From then on, he didn't really need massage to rid him of backache, but it had become a part of the couple's program, which both of them considered one of the best parts of the day.

If you're strong enough to press hard in a clumsy position, you may be able to milk out those backache-causing acids for yourself. Here's the technique:

Solution 8

1. Sit on a straight chair.
2. If practical, bare your back and lubricate with mineral oil. (This makes it easier, but you can still get some relief massaging through a layer of cloth.)
3. Ball both hands into fists. Lean forward and reach around with both arms to press the backs of your knuckles into your back muscles as high up as you can reach.
4. Continuing pressure, slide your knuckles down to the base of your spine.
5. Repeat several times, until your backache disappears.

Simple as it seems, this method saved Perry T.'s job. As a clerk in a theater ticket bureau, Perry was on his feet all day, having to be nice to the customers. And by the end of the day, with his back hurting like a toothache, he just didn't have any patience. He came to my office in desperation after his boss had told him he'd be fired if he barked at one more client.

I showed Perry how to milk acids out of his back muscles with the back of his knuckles, and he agreed to give it a try. A few months later, I needed tickets for a play, and Perry waited on me. It was late in the day, but he still wore a big smile.

Perry told me that he had worn out two shirts rubbing through them before he bought new ones with slick, tightly-woven fabric. But he figured it was worth it. With instant relief from back pain available whenever it started to bug him, his smile stayed big from morning to night. And his pay packet had gotten bigger, too; his boss recognized his cheerful mien with a nice raise.

Whenever I talk to patients about massage, they bring up the subject of machines. None of the vibrators I've seen have enough punch to milk waste products out of your big back muscles. But you may be able to get enough impact from spurts of water, using this approach:

<u>Solution 9</u>

1. Remove any flow-restriction devices from your shower, and install a head with capacity to deliver firm pulsations.

2. Adjust the temperature toward the hot side (heat helps to relax the muscles, so that their tension doesn't block milking action of pulse impact).

3. Drape a towel over your back so that the shower comes through it. (That holds the heat and makes it more effective.)

4. Stand with both knees bent and both hands resting on your knees, with the pulsating shower striking through the towel to the sore muscles.

5. Move your hips as if you were drawing figure 8s with your rectum, so that the muscles alternately contract and relax.

6. Continue for about 10 minutes (if the hot water holds out).

Sitting, standing, and working—all of these positions can make your back hurt. But you've found effective remedies for all those varieties. Here's a quick review:

SECTION ONE'S KEY POINTS

If you get back pain at the base of your neck when you drive long distances, firm, kneading massage gives instant relief. Shifting positions or using a pad to brace your head makes relief last longer.

Deep, kneading massage milks out the lactic acid that

over-activity leaves in your muscles. When your bigger back muscles hurt, the pressure needed can be substantial. You may need to "roll away the pain" with a tennis ball, softball, or firm rubber children's ball. If you have a strong helper, you can get relief with the type of massage described in Solution 7. Or you may be able to get relief with the knuckle self-massage described in Solution 8.

You can also drape a towel over your back and direct a hot, intensely pulsing shower through it.

SECTION TWO

SEVEN WAYS TO EASE BACK PAIN FROM TENSION

A tense muscle works hard and continuously. So a muscle that stays tight from nervous tension produces even more lactic acid than does one that contracts intermittently to lift heavy objects, because it produces irritants constantly.

If you get muscle pain from tension, you can use the same lactic acid removing methods which work so well for work-weary pain. But it's awfully hard to milk acids out of a muscle so tight that it feels like a board. "Rolling away the pain" and massage work much better if you get the muscles to loosen up first.

You'll find these special measures worthwhile if you get tension backache:

TENSION BACKACHE

What you feel:

Steady, dull back pain, usually all the way up the back and neck, sometimes with twinges extending around the left chest.

Cause:

Muscle spasm from nervous tension. The pain comes partly from lactic acid accumulation and partly from the pressure of tense, hard muscles against nerves.

Muscles which tension has put into spasm become so hard that it becomes almost impossible to milk acids out of them. You need to loosen up those muscles before you can milk away the irritating acids. One method uses localized heat. If you're handy with tools, you can easily make a back-baking chamber which directs light bulb heat[1] evenly across your whole back and use it according to these directions:

Solution 1

1. Obtain two 2-foot × 4-foot pieces of ½-inch plywood, two L braces, aluminum foil, cement or glue, four ceramic simple

[1]Light bulbs give off much more of their energy as infrared than as visible light. The infrared they develop is closer to the solar variety and better absorbed to heat tissue than is that developed by most "infrared lamps."

ceiling fixtures, 18-gauge two-strand wire, and a plug.

2. Fasten the 2-foot ends of the plywood together at right angles, forming a narrow tent. Measure along the peak of the "tent" and make marks 5 inches and 10 inches from each end. Measure down 6 inches from the peak from these marks, alternating sides. Drill 1-inch holes at these points.

3. Line the inside of the "tent" with aluminum foil, cementing same in place and cutting out the four holes.

4. Install the four ceiling fixtures to the inside of the "tent" adjacent to the holes, and wire them in parallel to the plug.

5. Put 100-watt bulbs in all four sockets.

6. Bare your back and lie underneath the "tent" (Figure 4). Check to see that the

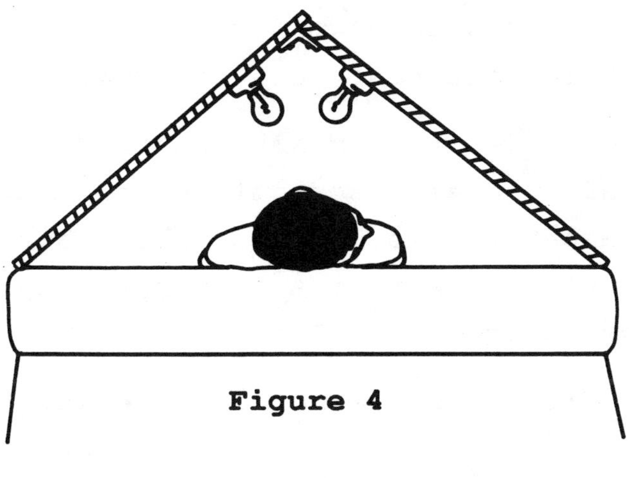

Figure 4

bulbs themselves are at least 1 foot away from your skin.

7. Plug in and enjoy the soothing warmth. If your skin gets too warm, unplug until the bulbs cool and unscrew one or more of them until it will not light. When you have adjusted the heat, enjoy it for 10 minutes or so.

8. Now try whichever of the "backache from overwork" solutions (4 to 9 in Section One) seems practical.

If you're not handy with tools, you can get similar effect with this technique:

Solution 2

1. Obtain two lamps with reflectors, such as gooseneck desk lamps, photographer's clamp-on lamps, or mechanic's trouble lights. Fit them with 100-watt bulbs.

2. Unless the reflectors are made of aluminum, line them with aluminum foil. This makes them reflect heat more effectively.

3. Bare your back and sit backward on a straight chair, straddling the back. Arrange the two lamps so that they shine on your low back from a distance of about 1 foot. (See Figure 5.)

4. For greater or lesser intense warmth, move closer or farther from the lights.

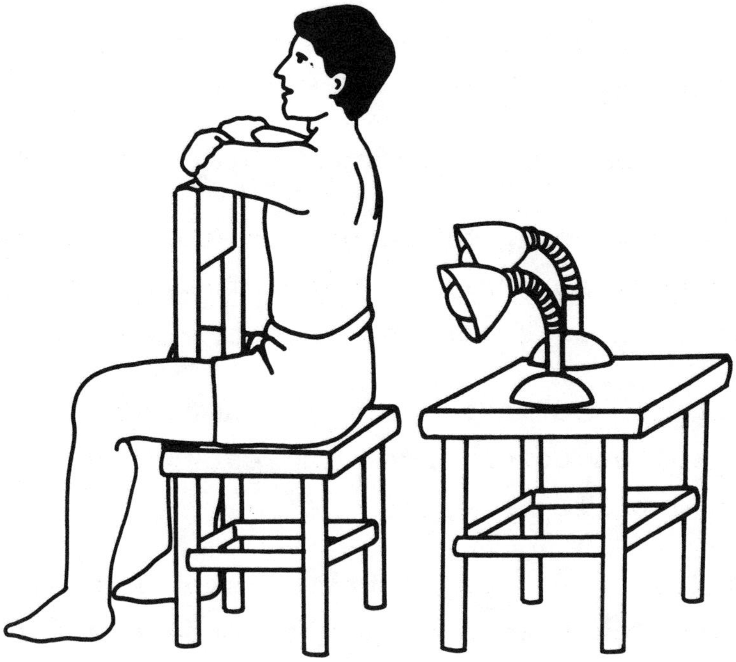

Figure 5

5. Enjoy the soothing warmth for 10 minutes or so.

6. Now try whichever of the "backache from overwork" Solutions (4 to 9 in Section One) seems practical.

When your back muscles are tense, chances are the muscles in the rest of your body are tense, also. Each one of the following three methods will help you to relax all the muscles in your body, including those in your back.

<u>Solution 3</u>

1. Set a timer for 45 minutes, in case you

fall asleep during this very relaxing routine.

2. Fill your tub with tepid water, about 92°F.

3. Tie a washrag or length of gauze to the faucet, so that the water runs down it instead of splashing into the pool.

4. Get in and make yourself comfortable, using a rolled towel under the back of your neck as a pillow.

5. Adjust the taps so that a slow stream of water at that same temperature constantly enters the tub (and leaves through the overflow drain).

6. Lie quietly in the tub, stirring only to avoid stiffness or discomfort, for 45 minutes. You will find that after the first half hour your body gradually relaxes completely.

The next two methods call for special equipment. You can usually get access to one type or the other at a local athletic facility or club.

Solution 4

1. Locate a whirlpool bath in a local athletic club or facility. Ideally, the temperature should be about 108°F, but you may have difficulty finding one that warm (since

children can be harmed by temperatures over 104°F).

2. Lie in the bath with streams of bubbles directed at your back and at other tense or uncomfortable muscles.

3. Continue for about 15 minutes.

Many health, athletic, tennis, and golf clubs, and even apartment complexes, have saunas. To get the full effect from a sauna, you need to follow the heat with cold. So if you have high blood pressure or some other condition which could be aggravated by cold applications, you'll have to use another method. Otherwise, you'll find that saunas can be very relaxing. Here's the technique:

Solution 5

1. Sit as high in the sauna as you can tolerate (higher gets hotter).

2. Splash water on the hot rocks occasionally to build heat.

3. Stay in the sauna until both your palms and the soles of your feet are sweating (usually about 10 minutes).

4. Go to the shower, and adjust it to maximum cold. As the cold water strikes each new skin area, you will gasp briefly.

5. You can decrease the gasp reflex by rubbing that area briskly as the water first strikes it.

6. After all areas have been exposed, the cold shower will feel like warm honey striking your skin. This happens because of the very brisk circulation of warm blood brought about by the prior heat.

7. While most "sauna addicts" think it's the heat that gives the benefit, that isn't true. What the sauna really does is let you tolerate cold showers or baths which you wouldn't be able to stand otherwise.

8. Continue the icy shower until you begin to feel the cold, usually about 5 minutes.

9. Towel off briskly, and proceed with whichever measures seem suitable from Section One's Solutions 4 to 9.

Sometimes the misery of tension-caused backache spreads beyond the back itself. If tense back muscles press against the nerves which follow your rib cage, you get pain which extends part way around your chest. You feel sharp twinges, mainly on the left (because your right arm tends to be supported by your desk, your grip on the steering wheel, etc.). You can quickly relieve the discomfort with this simple home remedy:

Solution 6

1. Sit sideways on a straight-backed chair with your right side against the back.
2. The top of the back should be about midway up your rib cage—if it is too high, sit on extra cushions.
3. Stretch your left arm straight up; then bend your elbow and touch your right ear.
4. Lean sideways against the chair back, and push your raised left elbow as far up and to the right as possible. You should feel this drawing your left ribs apart.
5. Hold this position for about 10 seconds, then stop stretching but remain in about the same position.
6. Rest for 10 seconds; then repeat.
7. Go through about ten such cycles.
8. If someone is willing to help you, he or she can increase the rib cage stretch by standing behind you, bracing the chair with his or her right hand and pressing your left armpit up and toward the chair back.

Larry P. had built a nice following as an accountant and tax preparer, but he wasn't sure he could continue in that career. Each of the seven years before I first saw him, he suffered through the tax season with chest pain. It would start about March first and stay with him until the middle of April.

Larry's other doctors listened to his heart and studied his cardiograms and then told him that nothing was wrong. But that wasn't enough to put his mind at rest. He knew that <u>something</u> was wrong or he wouldn't hurt. And he was so afraid that his stressful job was ruining his heart that he had put out feelers to find a different line of work, even though he had built a fine practice.

I listened to his heart and did a cardiogram, too. Once someone starts worrying about his heart, he needs to know those things are normal before he can possibly relax. Then I showed him how to do Solution 5's rib-stretching maneuver and helped him through his first few stretches.

His pain vanished instantly, which proved that pressure on intercostal nerve roots caused his problem; stretching wouldn't have done a thing for heart pain.

Larry keeps a straight-backed chair at his office now, specifically for rib-stretching use. As soon as tax season starts, he stretches four or five times a day, and the pain never even starts. And he still does my tax returns (along with about a thousand others) every year.

No one knows how to relax muscles without working hard at it. People (including doctors) who tell you to "just relax" don't understand the situation. But you can learn to loosen up tense muscles if you spend some time and effort on the following technique. You'll need to spend about half an hour a day for three or four weeks learning to use it, but the results (both in control of backache and in control of tension itself) more than justify the effort.

Solution 7

1. At first, you will need to remove all physical and mental distractions.
   - Lie down in a quiet, darkened room.
   - Support your lower legs and arms with pillows, keeping them level with the ground.
   - Close your eyes.
2. Now use the fact that you already know how to contract muscles to learn to relax them.
   - Hold your neck a little bit stiff, then moderately stiff, then very stiff, then as stiff as you can make it.
   - Now move back down that scale to very stiff, then to moderately stiff, then to a little stiff, then to normal.
3. Now go one step farther, relaxing the muscles beyond their normal state.

4. Practice this several times, until you have the feel of loosening up a muscle beyond its normal "resting" state.

5. Now try to do the same with the muscles of your right shoulder, then your right upper arm, lower arm, then hand.

6. Continue around your whole body, relaxing muscle groups in your right leg, left leg, left arm, back, abdomen, face, and scalp.

7. When you have relaxed every muscle group in your body, take time out for three deep breaths. Then start around again, relaxing each muscle group a bit further than you left it last time around.

8. Continue for about 20 minutes, by which time you should feel thoroughly relaxed.

9. If you follow this method at least once a day for three weeks, you will find yourself more and more able to relax muscles at will. At this point, you can use this new capacity (without the dark room, pillows, etc.) to loosen up back muscles sufficiently to use the methods described in Section One's Solutions 4-9 to relieve your back pain.

You can carry the progressive muscular relaxation method one step farther to stave off most tension-generated physical complaints. Do this with the "refresher slouch," as follows:

Solution 8

1. Sit in a straight chair with both feet on the ground.
2. Put both hands on your knees.
3. Let your head slump forward onto your chest.
4. Now relax each of your body parts in succession, going "around", then "up." Relax
   - your right shoulder, upper arm, forearm and hand
   - your right thigh, lower leg, and foot
   - your left thigh, lower leg, and foot
   - your left shoulder, upper arm, forearm, and hand
   - your abdominal muscles
   - your lower back
   - your upper back
   - your neck
   - your face and forehead
   - your scalp
5. Take a deep breath and start another go-round. Continue for about 2 minutes.

If you follow this routine several times a day,

particularly whenever you begin to feel muscle tension building up, you will find that many of the tension-generated backaches (and other discomforts) which have plagued you will disappear, just as Peter K.'s did.

Peter worked as an airplane mechanic when I first met him. But he really wanted to fly. Over the years, he had spent every dime he could spare and countless hours taking lessons and building airtime. But he couldn't even think of getting a commercial pilot's license because of the pills he took for back pain. Even muscle relaxants would have made him ineligible, and the strong tranquilizers he had sometimes taken (Librium and Valium) would have made the Federal Aviation Administration (FAA) flip.

I explained progressive muscular relaxation and the refresher slouch to Peter.

A few months later he told me that he hadn't really believed that he could throw his tranquilizers and muscle relaxants away when he had been on one product or another for years. But he gave it an all-out try. At first, he spent half an hour every day in a darkened bedroom. Then he found himself able to relax by slouching in a chair. Finally, he learned to do most of his relaxing in odd moments, while waiting for traffic lights to change or holding on the telephone. But he hadn't taken a relaxant or tranquilizer since learning the progressive muscular relaxation method.

In his pill-free state he had passed his FAA Class I examination, and his boss had recommended him for a pilot job.

If you're on a 747 and notice that the pilot slumps in his seat every spare moment, maybe it's Peter. He's been flying those monsters for three years now.

SECTION TWO'S KEY POINTS

You can treat or prevent the backaches which come with nervous tension in several ways. You need to loosen up tense, hard muscles before you can use the above methods to milk acids out of them. Light bulb heat, continuous tubs, whirlpool baths, or saunas all can do the trick.

If tight muscles press a nerve against a rib, pain may shoot part way around your chest. Stretching exercises will instantly relieve it.

Nobody can just "relax" without learning how. Spend a few minutes a day for a few weeks mastering this technique. You'll be repaid many times over in freedom from muscle pain and in improved efficiency.

SECTION THREE

HOME REMEDIES FOR BACK STRAINS AND SPRAINS

When you strain or sprain your back, sometimes you don't realize at first how badly you are hurt. Your foot slips while you're carrying a heavy object, and you twist suddenly to keep from falling. Maybe you just get the sensation that something has snapped or clicked in your back, with no real pain at all.

A few moments later your back begins to hurt. It hurts more and more. The muscles tighten up, usually mainly on one side. You walk tilted to the side (and wish you didn't have to walk at all, because every movement hurts). Then you know you're in for a siege of trouble.

What you feel:

At first, a snap or crunch in your back, perhaps with just a twinge of pain. Later, increasing steady back pain, generally concentrated on one side.

Cause:

Stretched or torn ligaments just behind the facet joints in your spine. Each of your vertebrae has four of these joints adjacent to your spinal canal, two of which flexibly link it with each of its neighbors. A strain or sprain involves stretching or tearing of the ligaments which support those joints. This stretch or tear makes the blood and lymph vessels in those ligaments leak irritating material, including blood and lymph, which cause pain when loose in your tissues. Your body must carry away this irritating material before the pain will subside.

If you take action right away, half an hour or so devoted to care for the injury can cut the discomfort you're due to suffer in half. You can quickly **shrink up the leaking vessels**, so that they spew out less irritant. Here's the technique:

Solution 1

1. Fill a plastic bag with ice cubes.
2. Wet a towel with cold water, and wring out the excess.
3. Lie on your stomach, with clothing pulled away from the lower back area.
4. Lay the wet towel across the injured area. Put the ice bag on top.
5. Chill the area thoroughly for at least 20 minutes.
6. If the cold becomes too intense, put

another wet towel between the ice bag and your skin.

7. Back pain may develop during this treatment. That's the pain we're trying to minimize, which would have been worse (and lasted longer) without the cold.

8. If pain becomes worse shortly after you stop chilling the area, chill it again immediately.

9. Otherwise, chill for 10 to 20 minutes three or four times a day for two or three days, depending on the severity of the injury (which you'll be able to evaluate when the pain develops to its full extent).

When you chill the injured part promptly, you shrink the area's blood and lymph vessels. That cuts down the amount of irritant which leaks into your tissues from torn ligaments. Free blood or lymph irritates tissue, causes pain and muscle spasm, and delays recovery. So prompt chilling really helps.

Cy P.'s case was a good example. At age 55, Cy usually hired a neighbor's son to shovel snow for him. But when 10 inches fell on a Saturday and the boy wasn't around, Cy got out his shovel. His foot slipped on an icy patch while he was heaving away the heavy snow the county plow had bladed into the end of his drive. He felt something snap in his back, and the pain began building up.

Cy had reservations for a skiing trip the next week, which he had been planning for months. So he called me right away, hoping he could keep the back strain from ruining his trip. Having suffered several back strains before, he knew he wouldn't be well in a week without special measures.

With all that snow right at hand, I suggested that he put some in a plastic garbage bag and chill down the injured area immediately. He seemed amazed at the idea; until he called, he had planned a hot shower. But he went along with the idea and chilled—10 minutes on, 10 minutes off—for about an hour.

Cy did come into my office later and I strapped him up, exactly the way I'll describe in Solution 2. He told me later that he pulled the tape off himself up at Aspen. Although most people with back strains find that each attack gets worse and lasts longer, thanks to prompt chilling, Cy's had stayed mild and lasted only half as long as any of the previous episodes.

What if you miss the moment—if you don't realize that

you've been badly hurt until spasm-generated pain develops?

Chilling still helps, and should be your top priority for 48 hours. Bleeding into tissue continues for some time after an injury, and you can do at least a little good by limiting it anywhere along the line. Here's the succession of events you need to fight:

1. Torn blood and lymph vessels leak irritating fluid into the tissues.
2. Muscle spasm occurs, induced partly by movement of the torn tissue and partly by irritation from leaked-out fluids.
3. Pain from the muscle spasm causes more muscle spasm and then more pain.
4. This vicious circle of pain causing spasm and spasm causing pain continues to build discomfort and distress.

Along with control of leakage from torn vessels, your first step in curing back strain is to brace the area to prevent continued motion at the site of the torn fibers. Here's how:

Solution 2

1. You will need a willing helper, a roll of 2-inch cloth adhesive tape, a razor, some tincture of benzoin (obtainable without

prescription at any drugstore), and scissors.

2. Lie on your stomach on a firm surface with a pillow under your chest and another under your knees to increase the hollow in your lower back.

3. Get your helper to strap your back, following these directions:

    - Shave the area from the bottom half of your rib cage to your hips.
    - Apply tincture of benzoin to this area and let it dry (almost instantaneous).
    - Smoothly apply a piece of tape diagonally from your left hip to your right flank, passing just above the crease between your buttocks (Figure 6).
    - Apply a crossing piece of tape from your right hip to your left flank.
    - Apply overlapping parallel strips up your back to the level of the bottom of your shoulder blades.
    - Apply pieces of tape longitudinally along the cut ends of the various pieces of tape, to help keep them from working loose.

Strapping which holds your back in a tilted-back

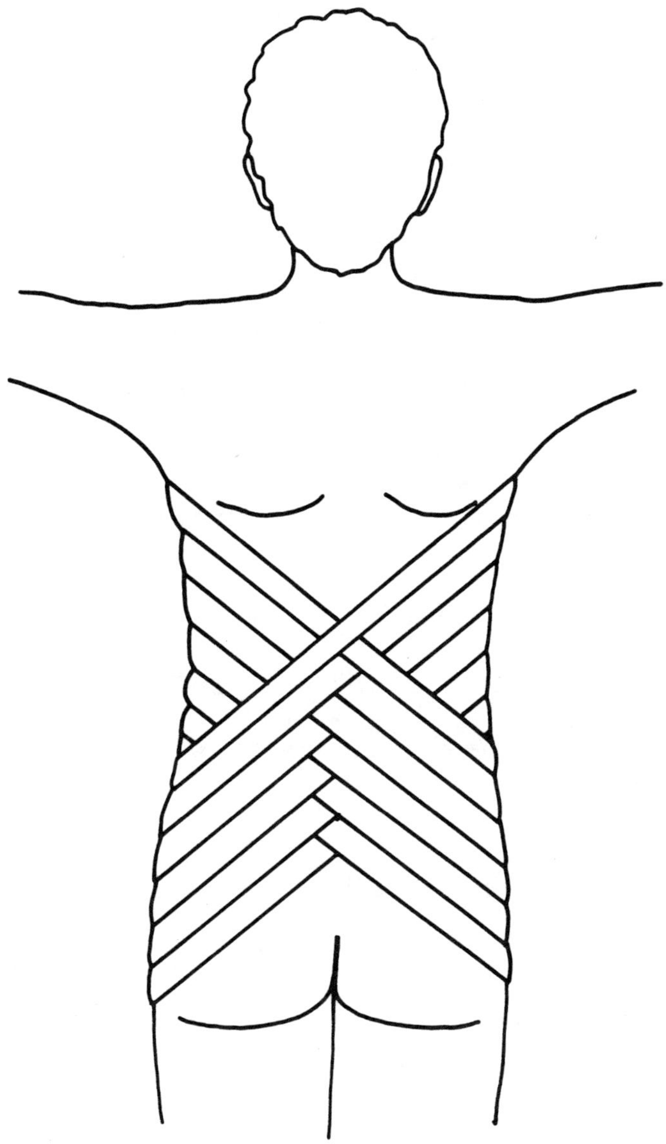

Figure 6

position takes the strain off the injured ligaments. You should leave this in place for about ten days, using sponge baths instead of showers or tubs.

If you still need to chill the injured area, you can do so right through the tape. Just apply your ice bag directly, without an intervening wet towel. If you need to temper the cold, put several layers of plastic instead of extra towels between your ice bag and the tape.

When your helper goes to remove the tape, a series of sharp jerks hurts less than slow, steady pull. If your back still hurts more without the support than with it, get your helper to reapply the strapping.

Meanwhile you can take aspirin to combat inflammation and spasm as well as for pain relief. Aspirin will help break the vicious spasm-pain-more spasm circle.

Solution 3

1. Don't "tough it out." Pain relief actually speeds healing besides giving temporary relief. Adequate amounts of aspirin speed recovery as well as relieve pain.

2. You may have some concern about the risk of internal bleeding from aspirin. Small doses of aspirin (half an adult tablet or 2½ grains) keep your body from forming one of a pair of opposing enzymes important to clotting. If you continue to take aspirin until the supply of that enzyme is exhausted, it will "thin your blood." But larger doses actually reverse this effect. Large doses inhibit the formation of both enzymes, keeping them still in balance. So

high aspirin doses have less effect on clotting than do small ones.

3. If you have some special reason to fear any impairment in clotting, such as history of bleeding ulcer, you should probably get a different pain- and spasm-fighting medicine (probably by seeing a doctor, since effective alternative preparations are only available by prescription). Otherwise, the doses suggested below will very rarely cause any problem.

4. Proper aspirin dosage depends on your ideal rather than your actual body weight. Aspirin doesn't penetrate into your fat cells. Excess fat doesn't affect the concentration of aspirin in the other tissues or the rate at which your body disposes of it.

   - If you should weigh 100 to 140 pounds, take two 5-grain aspirin tablets four times a day, after each meal and at bedtime.
   - If you should weigh 141 to 180 pounds, take three tablets.
   - If you should weigh over 180, take four tablets.

5. In this situation, you're using aspirin to combat inflammation and spasm as well as for pain relief. So you should take it on

schedule whether or not you have pain—"by the day" instead of "by the dose."

6. If you get ringing in your ears or dizziness (showing that you are more sensitive to the effects of aspirin than most people), cut back to half the recommended doses.

7. Take the appropriate amount for at least three days.

8. When you begin to wonder whether you need it any more, cut the dose in half and take it for at least two more days.

9. Don't quit entirely until you feel virtually well.

When Joe and Mary P.'s car got stuck in a rut on their way to a party, Joe figured that as a hefty 40-year-old truck driver, he ought to be able to move it himself. He did move the car, but only after something snapped in his back. It didn't hurt too badly at first, especially since the party involved considerable beverages thought to kill pain. But by the next morning he could hardly get out of bed.

That afternoon, I saw him in my office. He walked in tilted to the right, and the muscles in his lower back were tight and hard from spasm. When I pressed the tip of my thumb into several spots, I found one which made him wince. Everything pointed to an ordinary backstrain, so I strapped Joe's back, using exactly the same method described in Solution 2, and told him to take aspirin "by the day, not by the dose." When he returned a week later, he was well.

FIGHTING MUSCLE SPASM

When you strain your back, a large part of your pain comes from muscle spasm. Spasm causes pain two different ways:

- By stimulating pain nerves inside the muscle itself

- By accumulating lactic acid through sustained contraction, causing painful irritation of tissue.

You can take action against each of these causes of pain from muscle spasm.

Solution 4

1. You'll find that you need sleep or rest and that very firm support helps you to get it.
2. Fill a 1-gallon Ziploc® storage bag with dry sand.

3. Put it inside another plastic bag in case of leaks.

4. If you sleep on a firm mattress, put the bag of sand under your lower back.

5. If you usually use a water bed or soft mattress, lie on the floor with the sand bag under your lower back. This will take the "stretch" off tight muscles and make them hurt less.

6. As an alternate position, you can lie on your stomach with the sandbag and several pillows under your chest and head to arch your back.

When you want to get up out of bed, you'll find that your usual way of getting to an upright position causes severe back pain. Here's how to avoid that discomfort:

Solution 5

1. Before you try to get out of bed, lie on your side near the edge. Fold the leg closest to the mattress up against your chest and grasp your knee with both hands. Pull that knee as close to your chest as possible.

2. While holding one leg in this position, roll up onto your fanny by making appropriate movements with the other leg.

3. When both feet are flat on the floor, let

go of your knee. Place both hands on top of the lower part of your thighs. With your arms rigid, rock forward to put your weight on your feet.

4. Walk your hands up your thighs, moving one at a time, to brace your back while you straighten up.

You'll also find that it helps to mobilize the lactic acid which accumulates from the constant contraction of spastic muscle. It's hard to do this with ordinary massage, even using the closed-fist technique described in Section One's Solution 6. But if someone helps you to "roll away the pain" with a method resembling Section One's Solution 4, moving out the accumulated lactic acid eases pain considerably.

Solution 6

1. You'll need a helper and the same equipment used in Section One's Solution 4. Use a tennis ball rather than a larger or softer one to overcome the hardness of the spastic muscle.

2. Get your helper to "roll away the pain" starting at the upper end of the spastic muscles.

3. When your helper gets to the injured area, he or she may find one spot which is very

tender. If so, he or she should avoid that spot on future passes.

4. Continue for 10 or 15 minutes, and repeat three times a day.

Since only part of your back pain in these circumstances is due to lactic acid, you won't get complete relief. But removal of the irritant will lessen both pain and spasm, which will help you to get well fast.

"CRICKS" AND "TWINGES"

Finally, let's consider those back injuries too mild to be called "back strain"—the "cricks" and "twinges." These generally come from a stretched ligament without broken blood vessels, but it never hurts to ice the area down. Some "cricks" which seem mild at first still involve enough bleeding into tissue to set up the irritation-spasm-pain-more spasm vicious circle.

If the pain hasn't become worse in 4 hours, you can be fairly sure no vessels have been breached. Then a hot compress usually gives relief. Here's the technique:

Solution 7

1. Fill a basin with water at 112°F (measured with a candy thermometer or another immersible, easily read variety). If you

don't have a suitable thermometer, make the water more than lukewarm, but considerably less than "as hot as you can stand it."

2. Fold a towel four to eight layers thick and dip in the water.

3. Place this over the sore area.

4. Cover with a dry towel to help hold the heat.

5. Wet the hot towel again every few minutes to keep it hot.

6. Continue about 20 minutes.

This usually controls the "crick" without need for other treatment. If it doesn't, consider the condition a strain or sprain instead of a "crick" and use the treatment methods described above.

Some of these "cricks" happen in vertebrae to which ribs attach instead of in your lower back. That's what happened to Zack K., for instance. As a 34-year-old golf course maintenance man, part of Zack's job was chopping sod with a machete. While whacking away, he got a sudden pain right between his shoulder blades. The pain felt like a cramp, with some aching or burning—hard to describe. It centered slightly to the left of his spinal column and didn't get worse with a deep breath or cough.

It didn't shoot around his chest or feel like it was piercing through.

All these qualities fit with a "slipped facet," which is just a fancy name for a crick in your back. Zack twisted one of the minor spine joints (called "facets") just enough to pop it out for a moment, without tearing or stretching any ligaments. He put heat on it for a few minutes three times that day, and the pain had vanished by morning. Zack used hot towels, but a hot shower through a towel or light bulb heat would have worked equally well.

SECTION THREE'S KEY POINTS

Prompt chilling cuts both the pain and the duration of any backstrain. Use an ice bag, snow, towels wet with water from a drinking fountain—whatever you can get <u>fast</u> to cool the tissue and shrink its leaking blood vessels.

Torn fibers around a facet joint cause some of your pain. Blood and lymph leaked into tissue irritate further. These factors cause muscle spasm, which causes a vicious circle of pain-spasm-more pain.

If you keep leakage of blood to a minimum with cold, movement of the torn fibers to a minimum with strapping, and pain to a minimum with aspirin, spasm usually decreases. Extra back arching with sandbag support and "rolling away" lactic acid from the tight muscles may also help.

Milder "cricks" in the back yield to heat. They can occur in the upper as well as the lower spine and shouldn't be confused with serious disease.

SECTION FOUR

SIX WAYS TO GET RELIEF FROM SPINAL ARTHRITIS

The facet joints in your spine can get sore and inflamed, just like any other joints in your body. For the weight they carry, they're very small—about as big as those in your thumb. You have a lot of them: two for every one of your vertebrae! So it's no wonder they cause a lot of misery when arthritis hits them.

Pain usually starts gradually. It may involve your upper, lower, or entire spine. Usually it gets worse whenever the barometric pressure drops (which gives you an unfortunate way of predicting the weather).

You generally hurt the most when you wake up in the morning, feel better after you've moved around a bit, then become more sore as you get tired in the evening (but never quite as sore as you are when you first wake up).

SLEEP SUPPORT

Since the morning misery seems related to sleep support, that's the first element you should attack.

Solution 1

Sleep on a superfirm surface. When you sleep on a soft mattress, it molds to your body. Your breathing motions and minor body movements don't cause the slightest motion in spinal joints. This lets those joints "freeze" into the painful stiffness of morning misery.

A very firm sleeping surface helps by making your body rather than your mattress shift with these movements. (Perhaps it also helps by making your sleep a bit more restless—every time you shift positions you move some of those stiff joints.)

A Japanese sleeping mat (futon) on the floor accomplishes this end beautifully.

Second choice: a cotton mattress (generally sold mainly in camp cot size) or a thin, firm sponge rubber mattress on a piece of ¾-inch plywood on top of your innerspring mattress. Cover all the plywood's cut edges with adhesive tape to avoid getting splinters under your nails while making the bed.

Sometimes you need to trade part of your sleeping comfort for morning relief. Alice P. had to make such a trade, for instance. When her back first started to hurt at age 55, she bought a water bed. By turning the heat regulator all the way up, she made that unit into a giant hot pad, which made her back feel better when she first lay down. But morning stiffness got worse and worse over the next three years. She told me that it felt just like someone boring into the back of her chest with a big auger. And the pain would last for two or three hours, no matter what medicine she took.

When Alice told me about this, I remembered that she had bought a hospital bed while nursing her husband through his last illness. That bed had a very firm mattress. So I suggested she try sleeping on it for a few nights.

She also started to use the other methods we're going to discuss. But even with all of them working for her, she still found that she needed firm sleep support. Every time she tried to go back to her water bed, morning stiffness returned to plague her. After six months, she gave up and replaced the water bed. With firm sleep support and the other measures, she totally avoided morning stiffness.

Alice wouldn't have gotten well just by changing her bedding. She needed medication, too.

IBUPROFEN AND ASPIRIN

Of the medications available without a prescription, ibuprofen usually proves best. I've used the generic name rather than the brand name to save you money. You've heard of Advil and Motrin, the names under which this medicine was originally distributed. Now several other companies make and market ibuprofen under their own trade names. These "generics" cost considerably less—$3.06 for 50 as opposed to $5.76 at one drugstore—for the same amount of the same medication.

<u>Solution 2</u>

1. When using ibuprofen to fight inflammation rather than for temporary pain relief, always take it on schedule instead of waiting until you hurt. You get best results if you "hit it hard" and then taper off.

2. Start with four tablets every eight hours (twelve a day). This sounds like a lot, but the prescription form of the same medicine is twice as strong as the ones you can buy over the counter. So twelve a day only amounts to twice the minimum effective inflammation-fighting dose.

3. If you have a sensitive stomach, always take food or milk with ibuprofen. The most common side effects are nausea and heartburn, which happen much less often if the medicine merges with acid-neutralizing proteins in your stomach.

4. Unless you get side effects, continue the full dose for three days, or until your pain disappears.

5. Then taper the dose one tablet per day. Decrease the morning dose before the afternoon one, and the afternoon one before the evening one (which helps stave off "morning misery"). Continue to reduce the dose day by day until you begin to get twinges again or until you reach six per day (two per dose).

Mabel S. worked in amateur theater for years before getting a lead part. So she tried to "grin and bear it" when her back began to hurt two weeks before opening night. She took an aspirin or Tylenol tablet every now and then, but it didn't seem to help. Finally she decided that she just couldn't cavort around the stage with every muscle in her back rock-hard and painful. So she came to me for help.

Mabel's temperature was 99°F, and she really should have been in bed. But with the play coming up, we decided to give ibuprofen a chance. After the first day's heavy dose, she felt somewhat better but not well. We kept the dose high one more day, then tapered down. Five days later, the play opened, and Mabel made it a hit. She still got a little stiff in the mornings at that point, but after another week she felt fully well.

At normal drugstore prices, even generic ibuprofen is costly, and you might need the medicine for weeks, months, or years. If you have health insurance or a Medicare supplement which covers prescription medications, you'll save a lot of money if you ask your doctor to prescribe ibuprofen or an equivalent preparation. Remember that the prescription form is stronger, so you should take only the number of pills specified on the label.

Ibuprofen has two advantages over aspirin for long-term use. First, if you're taking half an aspirin a day to avoid coronary disease (like most doctors, including me), more aspirin will decrease instead of increase the blood-thinning effect (see Solution 3 in Section Three). Second, the greater chance of internal bleeding, although slight with the recommended doses, is enough to tip the balance.

On the other hand, aspirin costs a lot less. It may work without side effects even if you get nausea or heartburn from ibuprofen. And either ibuprofen or aspirin may give relief when the other doesn't work. So you may want to use aspirin according to this plan:

Solution 3

1. As a replacement for ibuprofen (never along

with it), take aspirin at the doses advised in Solution 3 of Section Three for three days.

2. If full doses give relief, cut back one tablet a day until you reach eight per day (two per dose).

3. If you get heartburn or nausea, try coated aspirin (Ecotrin or a generic equivalent). These tablets don't dissolve until they have passed through your stomach, which may solve the problem.

4. If your ears ring or if you get dizzy, this shows that you react unusually strongly to aspirin, so that smaller doses will work well for you. You'll usually get good results without side effects if you take half the usual dose.

5. If at any time you pass black, tarry stools (which may mean internal bleeding), stop aspirin and check with your doctor.

6. As with ibuprofen, aspirin works best if you hit the disorder hard, then taper off, instead of creeping up on the right dose. And also if you take it regularly to fight inflammation instead of waiting until you have pain.

PARAFFIN BATHS

Heat in any form seems to give some relief from arthritic

back pain, but the form which works absolutely best is the paraffin bath.

Solution 4

1. If you have heavy hair on your back, shave the area before your first treatment.
2. Heat 2 pounds of paraffin (from the canning supply section of your food store) with 1 pint of mineral oil (from your drugstore) in a double boiler.
3. When the paraffin has melted, remove from heat and let cool until a scum forms on top.
4. With a rubber-base paintbrush, apply several coats of the hot paraffin on the sore part of your back.
5. Cover with a dry towel.
6. Enjoy the soothing warmth for about 20 minutes.
7. Peel off the paraffin-oil mixture and put it back in the pan. You can use the same mixture many times.
8. After several treatments, you may want to apply slightly more intense heat. If so, change the proportion of paraffin to mineral oil. The less mineral oil you put in the mixture, the warmer it will be at the time of application. Try 2 pounds of paraffin with half a pint of mineral oil.

After trying this several times, if you want an even warmer application use straight paraffin with no mineral oil at all.

9. Always let the mixture cool until a scum forms. Don't try to make it hotter by short-changing the cooling phase, or you might get burned.

Sometimes I wondered if Mrs. R. would make it into my office. Past attacks of arthritis had twisted her fingers and locked up her knees, so that she walked with two canes. At age 62 the pain shifted mainly to her back.

On her first visit, I noticed red blotches on her arms. It turned out that she kept bees, especially so that she could get them to sting her. Over the years, she had found bee stings actually relieved her arthritis. (If you aren't allergic to them, they actually do provide useful protein inoculations. But at what a price in pain!). So I felt quite gratified a few weeks later when she told me that paraffin baths gave so much relief that she had disposed of the bees. The old deformities persisted, of course. But ultimately she got down to two or three paraffin baths a week, and still stayed free of pain.

ALTERNATE BACK-WARMING METHODS

You need someone to help you with paraffin baths. So

you may need to settle for another form of soothing warmth.

You can use light bulb heat with a back-baking chamber (Solution 1, Section Two) or lamps with reflectors (Solution 2, Section Two). Start your day with 10 minutes of soothing warmth, then follow up with a warm shower. This routine usually thoroughly relieves morning stiffness.

If you aren't handy with tools, your best choice may be a heating pad. I've made this a last choice because heating pads have major disadvantages. Pads with circulating water cost a lot, and those with wires give uneven heat. But they do give considerable comfort, if the better warming methods aren't available.

Solution 5

1. The best kind of heating pads pump thermostatically controlled water through passages in a rubber pad. This keeps the heat even and safe, even if you lie on top of the pad.

   These units cost much more than an ordinary pad, so you may want to rent one for a week to see whether it gives enough relief to make one worth buying.

These units can be found in hospital supply stores if unavailable at your drugstore.

2. If you use an ordinary heating pad with imbedded electric wires, keep the control set at "low." Crossing wires, or wires which get too close to each other because of wrinkles or folds in the pad, can cause hot spots to reach dangerous levels at the higher settings.
3. Never lie on top of an electric heating pad, because the heat can build up until it burns you.

USING GENTLE MASSAGE

Proper massage often helps to relieve arthritic back pain. Gentle stroking moves lymph out of the passages into which fluid from congested joints must move. (The deep, lymph-mobilizing kneading you use for work-weary muscle aches won't work here. The spine's joints lie too deep, and they are located in hard, unyielding tissue.)

Solution 6

1. Lie on your stomach on a firm surface which your helper can easily reach without bending.
2. Get your helper to lubricate your back with mineral oil.
3. He or she should use the surfaces of all

four fingers on each hand and both palms and should stroke gently and rhythmically from the base of your spine toward your head. Each stroke should be 10 to 12 inches long. It should begin and end with very light pressure, with mild but distinct pressure during the midstroke.

4. Every stroke should begin and end ½ to 1 inch or so farther toward your head.

5. This pattern should be repeated two or three times.

6. Then your helper should clean off the oil with rubbing alcohol.

Finally, there are some forms of spinal arthritis which need a doctor's care. We'll talk about that further in the last section of this report.

SECTION FOUR'S KEY POINTS

Arthritis can involve all or any part of your spine. You usually suffer most when you first get up in the morning. A stiff sleeping surface helps relieve this misery.

Ibuprofen often helps. It gets the nod over aspirin, but the decision is close. Whichever you use, start with a big dose, take the medicine regularly (not just when you hurt), and taper gradually to find the least amount which sustains the relief.

Heat also helps. Paraffin baths give the most relief. Light bulb heat or a heating pad help somewhat.

Gentle, stroking massage gives relief. Use it rather than the kneading type.

SECTION FIVE

HOW TO KEEP YOUR BACKBONE STURDY

Forty-six-year-old Harriet S. went to the laundromat feeling perfectly well. But when she started to carry her basket of wet wash from in front of the washing machine to the dryer, pain hit between her shoulder blades. It felt as if someone had shot her with an arrow.

She went home and laid down, which gave some relief. But the pain resumed when she stood up, and really shot through her when she coughed or sneezed.

What happened to Harriet? One of her vertebrae had collapsed from its normal blocklike shape into a wedge. This happened because of osteoporosis, which had thinned and weakened the internal structure of the vertebrae. Osteoporosis occurs when your body leaches calcium out of your bones. That calcium loss can result from too little calcium in your diet or from excess calcium loss through your kidneys or bowel. It thins all your bones, but your vertebrae, wrists, and hips have the least spare strength. So osteoporosis causes those bones to fracture with only minor injury—even just ordinary lifting in the case of the spine.

Harriet's condition was worse than most, but two out of every five women over age 40 have some sign of osteoporotic bone thinning. Men get this disorder, too, but usually at a somewhat older age.

Harriet spent the next week in bed. Then she gradually mobilized herself over the next two weeks. She had to lie down for 15 minutes every 2 or 3 hours for about 2 months before the pain left.

Then she started the preventive measures I'm going to explain. I was afraid she might have one or two more collapsed vertebrae before they took hold. But luckily she hasn't had any further trouble.

DETERMINING YOUR PRONENESS TO OSTEOPOROSIS

Should you be taking steps to avoid all this?

Here's how you can find out how prone you are to osteoporosis. First, determine your "personal proneness" score:

Traits	Problem	Evaluation	Score
Sex	Women have higher risk	Females add 15	
Age	Bone absorption increases with age	Add 1 for each year above 40	
Blond?	Lighter complexion generally means more risk	Blonds add 20, other whites and Asian Americans 10, blacks 5	
Slight?	Delicate build is at risk (wrist circumference shows bone weight)	Add 20 if delicate build, 10 if medium, 0 with heavy frame	
Skin quality	Thin, transparent skin makes high risk	Add 20 if you can see small vein branches on the back of hands	
Past menopause	Unreplaced sex hormones cut new bone formation	Add 20 if past menopause (40 if ovaries removed early)*	
Diet	Lack of calcium, vitamins C & D hurt bone production	Add 20 if you eat no dairy products, 10 if you don't eat them at least twice daily	
		Your personal total	

*Women can skip this item if hormone lack has always been replaced by prescribed estrogen-progesterone tablets or shots. Score half if now replaced. Men only suffer hormone lack if testes removed or heavily irradiated (as for tumor). The "male menopause" doesn't count.

Interpret that score according to this list:

- Over 100: Extreme risk. Should take all measures described here, and consider hormone replacement (by your doctor).
- 80–100: Great risk. Follow all measures described here conscientiously.
- 50–80: Moderate risk. The mild measures in Solutions 1, 2, and 3 suffice.
- Under 50: Minimal risk. Follow only suggestions which fit readily into your lifestyle.

Mabel J. first came to me when she was 45. She was very attractive—natural blond hair, fine bones, and delicate skin. You could see even tiny vein branches on the back of her hand, and her wrists and ankles were very small.

I explained that, unless she took countermeasures, these characteristics made her likely to become bent and bowed when she grew older. Mabel knew exactly what I was talking about, because she had seen it happen to her mother, whom she said "just shriveled up before she was sixty."

Mabel and I went over the measures I'm going to explain to you, and she stuck to them rigorously. She's 68 now, still straight-backed and dainty, standing as tall as ever (her mother had lost 5 inches from her initially modest height).

Mabel used every one of the following measures conscientiously:

CALCIUM INTAKE

Your body needs more calcium than any other mineral. Your system uses your bones not only as rigid supports but also as a reservoir for this crucial substance. Your nerves and muscles need a certain amount of calcium to function. So if you don't absorb enough from your food to make up for what you lose, your body draws calcium out of your bones, even though this weakens them.

Eating foods which contain calcium in a form your body can readily absorb keeps this from happening.

Solution 1

1. Eat lots of dairy products. You need the calcium from four glasses of milk a day.
2. If you drink less milk:
    - Eat yogurt (equivalent ounce for ounce)

- Eat cottage cheese (twice the calcium per ounce)

3. Don't eat calcium-blotters or destroyers within an hour of your dairy products. Oxalic acid, contained in spinach, beet greens, and rhubarb, keeps calcium from soaking into your system. So does phytic acid, contained in beans and other legumes and whole wheat, unless combined with yeast. (Beans can also be soaked in water for several hours, with the water then discarded, to remove phytic acid.) High-fiber cereals also blot up calcium and carry it through your bowel.

4. Keep track of total milk, yogurt, and cottage cheese intake for one week. If your dairy product consumption falls short, get a supply of calcium lactate tablets (available without a prescription). For each omitted glass of milk or equivalent, take two calcium lactate tablets daily.

5. Avoid excessive vitamin D. You need 400 milligrams a day, which you will almost certainly get from enriched milk, butter, or margarine. Over 1,000 milligrams a day actually harms calcium absorption. Check the labels on any vitamin preparations (or calcium-vitamin combinations) you use to be sure you don't add more than 600 milligrams a day of vitamin D to what you're getting in natural food sources.

EXERCISE TO BUILD BONE SUBSTANCE

The above tips will ensure that you're getting enough calcium into your system. But getting your body to build bone substance out of that calcium is another matter.

Exercise seems to be the key. People who live sedentary lives get much more osteoporosis than their active neighbors. So it seems that even mild exercise stirs your body to make stronger bones.

Solution 2

1. Start with a 5-minute daily walk (if you haven't been getting any exercise at all).

2. Increase the duration and pace gradually until you are walking briskly for 20 minutes daily.

3. If walking makes your back hurt or doesn't work out for other reasons, try swimming. Since the water supports your body weight, you can meet your exercise need in this way when other forms of exercise cause discomfort.

Besides general body exercise, certain specific procedures help. These movements strengthen the muscles which support your spine:

Solution 3

1. Lie on your back. Grasp both knees and pull them toward your chest. Pull hard for 5 seconds.

2. While still on your back, put both legs out straight. Bring one knee up and pull it toward your chest with both hands, keeping the other leg entirely straight. Hold for 5 seconds. Repeat with the other leg.

3. Bend your knees until your feet are flat on the floor. Roll your hips forward by tilting your pelvis, which should press the small of your back against the floor. Hold for 5 seconds.

4. Bend knees and fold your arms across your chest. Raise your head and shoulders a few inches off the floor. Hold for 3 seconds.

5. With legs straight, arms flat at your sides, raise head and shoulders. Hold 3 to 5 seconds.

6. Fold your arms in front of your chest and bring your bent knees up close to them. Slowly straighten your legs, keeping your heels at the same height from the floor. Slowly return to starting position.

7. Bend your knees with feet flat on floor. Fold your hands behind your head. Press both elbows against the floor for 5 seconds.

8. Tuck your chin down against your chest.

Squeeze your shoulder blades together strongly for 5 seconds.

9. Roll over onto your stomach with a pillow underneath your chest. Keep your chin tucked down against your chest. Squeeze shoulder blades together firmly for 5 seconds.

As your muscles build up, you can do each exercise two, three, or four times.

DECREASING CALCIUM LOSS

I've left this method until last because it disrupts your life-style considerably. You'll probably use it only if you have a high-risk index or actual signs of osteoporosis.

Solution 4

1. Cut down on foods and beverages which make more calcium pass through into your urine. These include excess red meat, sugar, salt, chocolate, coffee, soft drinks, and processed meats.
2. Quit smoking, if you are a smoker.

IF PREVENTION FAILS

You may already have osteoporosis, or you may not follow a strict enough preventive program. It's hard to believe you need to change your life-style to ward off a subtle change like gradually weakening bones, but if you don't, you might suffer a collapsed vertebra some day.

What you feel:

Sudden pain at one specific level between your shoulder blades, which gets steadily worse the longer you stay out of bed.

Cause:

You have lost bone strength through osteoporosis. This has weakened the weight-bearing bodies of your vertebrae. One of those bodies has given way under the burden of your weight and crunched down from its normal boxlike shape to a wedge.

Unless you minimize the effect and prevent further vertebral collapse, the extra forward curvature of your spine will make your back bend into a hump. The crunching will make you shorter, and the downward shift of your rib cage will press your abdominal organs forward to give you a "pot belly." All these changes, which you've probably thought of as coming from "old age," actually stem from osteoporosis.

So what should you do if you get sudden pain at one level, usually between your shoulder blades?

You'll probably be able to feel or see an unevenness in the spacing or prominence of your backbone's knobs (Figure 7). That will tell you for sure which vertebra has collapsed and make it easier for you to follow this approach:

Solution 5

1. Go to bed.
2. Be sure your sleep surface is very firm. If it isn't, get a cotton mattress and a bed board to put on top.
3. Partly fill a sandwich-size Ziploc® bag with sand, exhausting the air before you seal it. Place inside a larger bag (as a precaution against leaks).
4. Put this under the sore vertebra, which makes your body weight tend to pull the compressed area apart. That relieves pain and reduces later deformity.
5. Stay in bed for a week or ten days, by

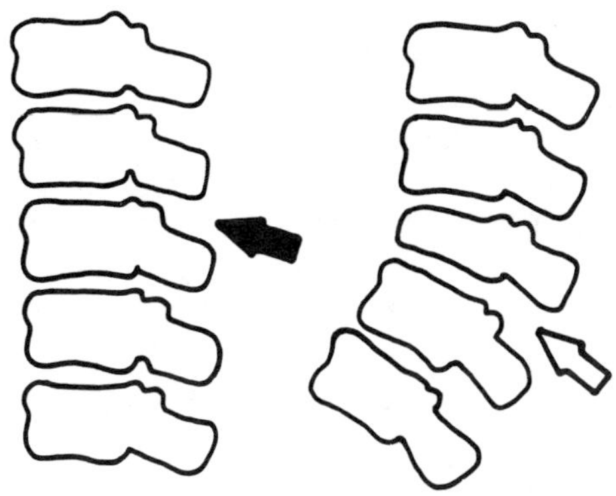

Figure 7

which time you should be able to stand up for a few minutes at a time.

6. Increase your "up" time, resting for a few minutes whenever the soreness increases, until healing is complete.

7. While in bed, do leg-vein-draining exercises every hour. Raise your feet as far as possible. With your ankle muscles loose, jiggle your feet rapidly for one minute.

8. Although this will usually prevent the main hazard of bed rest, which is leg-vein clots, you should also remain alert for this condition. Check every day (even after you are getting up some) for swelling of one or both ankles or tenderness in one or both calves. If either occurs, see your doctor right away.

Bed rest keeps pain to a minimum. It also may help to keep the damaged vertebra from collapsing further, perhaps to the point where nerve pressure occurs.

When you first get up, you may find that an abdominal binder helps prolong the interval before pain makes you go back to bed. An abdominal binder is a snug bandage which pushes in firmly on your abdomen. You can see for yourself what this does to your spine: Just sit in a straight chair and push firmly on your abdomen with both hands. See how your head moves up and back? That means the upper spine has straightened, taking stress off its front section—the very part which has given way when a vertebra crunches.

Solution 6:

1. Get an abdominal binder with Velcro® at your drugstore or hospital supply store.
2. If you prefer, cut and hem a piece of bleached muslin wide enough to cover your entire abdomen and long enough to overlap about 8 inches in the front. Use six or eight large safety pins to hold the latter snug.
3. Stand up. Take a deep breath and draw in your abdomen. Pull the binder tight while your stomach is flat and fasten it with the Velcro® or the pins.
4. Wear it under your clothes until bedtime.

As soon as you can do so comfortably, start the exercises described in Solution 3. These strengthen muscles which brace the injured area. They help both in easing the soreness and in minimizing deformity.

Once a vertebra has collapsed, you can't restore its original shape. If several collapse, you can lose inches of height and develop a bowed back with a protruding abdomen.

SECTION FIVE'S KEY POINTS

Two out of five American women over age 40 have osteoporosis. Men usually escape until an older age, but ultimately often suffer from this painful, deformity-causing disorder. But you don't need to ever have this condition.

If you're likely to get osteoporosis, a high score on this section's proneness test will warn you. Then you can increase your calcium intake. You can avoid foods that blot up calcium in your food and carry it through your system. You can take just the right amount of vitamin D—too much is worse than too little! You can exercise regularly and take specific spine-support-strengthening exercises. You can cut out caffeine and other materials which make your kidneys pour out extra calcium. If you smoke, you can quit smoking.

If one of your vertebrae crunches, you'll need to go to bed for a week and follow up with gradual mobilization using an abdominal binder and with special exercises.

Follow whatever measures your proneness level indicates. Then, at minimum cost to your life-style, you can live out your years with a painless, straight, full-length spine.

SECTION SIX

HOME REMEDIES FOR NERVE ROOT PRESSURE

If something touches the raw nerve in your tooth, you suffer severe pain. A ruptured or bulging disc presses on nerves ten times or more as large. You can see why it causes such agony!

HOW TO TELL DISC TROUBLES FROM ORDINARY BACK STRAIN

Since the measures you should use for ruptured or bulging discs differ completely from those appropriate for back strain, let's see how you can distinguish the two:

Feature	Back Strain	Ruptured Disc
Onset	Pain increases gradually	Sudden jolt of pain when nerve pressure occurs (sometimes days after initial injury)
Spread	As spasm develops, pain spreads from rib cage to hips	Shoots down leg, often to ankle
Character	Sharp ache	Agonizing jolt
Muscle spasm	Builds for 24 to 48 hours	Generally from start
Tenderness	One or more spots in back hurt with firm finger pressure	Sore area may hurt when touched (even gently) but no deep sore spots

Most of your weight rests on the stack of vertebral bodies with intervening discs. Discs rupture from too much pressure along the axis of your spine—the sudden jolt from the bottom if you're sitting on a toboggan that hits a bump, or the transmitted weight of something very heavy which you're trying to lift. At the time of injury, part of the firm ring at the margin of the disc breaks, but that tissue has no pain nerves. Pain starts when the gooey, soft cartilage within the disc pushes through the gap in the firm cartilage ring and presses on a nerve root. This may not occur immediately. You may feel nothing but a snapping sensation at the time of injury, with severe pain suddenly grabbing you hours or days later.

What you feel:

Sometimes a snapping sensation, then sudden stabbing or burning back pain. This often shoots down your leg, sometimes all the way to your ankle.

Cause:

Nerve pressure, usually from a ruptured or bulging disc.

No matter where pressure occurs along the course of a nerve, you feel the pain where that nerve ends. So pressure on nerve roots as they exit from the spinal canal can cause pain to shoot clear to your ankle. The most common cause of such pain is a ruptured or bulging disc.

The pads between your vertebrae have a gooey center surrounded by a firm ring of cartilage. The goo can burst through the ring or make it bulge to press against nerve roots. Such "ruptured" or "bulging discs" cause excruciating pain.

For example, Pete C. lifted a heavy object and felt something give way in his back. It didn't hurt much, and he didn't even report the accident to his foreman. Two days later he bent down to pull a weed in his garden, and pain shot through his back like a knife. He literally couldn't straighten up. He finally climbed hand over hand up the handle of his rake and hobbled into his house. By then, the pain had spread clear down his right leg, all the way to the ankle.

USING THE JACKKNIFE POSITION AND ASPIRIN

Pete needed a week to lessen his pain and muscle spasm. He took aspirin as described in Solution 3 of Section Three and followed this method:

Solution 1

1. Rent a hospital bed and bed pan.

2. Raise both the head and the knee support to about 45°.

3. Stay in bed in this "jackknife position" continuously until pain and spasm have substantially diminished. To make this method work, you have to stay in bed all the time. Every time you put your feet on the floor, you go back to square one. That's why you need the bed pan (and a lot of loving care).

4. The leg-vein-draining exercise advised in Solution 5 of Section Five can't be done in this situation, so it is important to have someone milk out the leg veins several times a day. Constant bed rest involves a definite risk of vein clots which this procedure helps to control.

   - Lubricate with mineral oil.
   - Make a ring around one ankle with both index fingers and thumbs.
   - Keeping moderate pressure on the entire circumference, slide this ring up the leg to the knee.
   - Repeat several times.
   - Follow the same procedure with the other leg.
   - Clean off the oil with rubbing alcohol.

5. The skin sensitivity which accompanies nerve root pain may make this procedure

uncomfortable, but you should tough it out if you can.

6. Also remain alert for puffiness or swelling of either ankle or new tenderness of the calf area, which might show that clots are forming. <u>If these occur, call your doctor.</u>

As with back strain, ruptured disc pain causes muscle spasm which then makes the situation worse. Take full doses of aspirin (Solution 3, Section Three) to control muscle spasm as well as pain.

If you relieve the muscle spasm, the goo that presses on the nerve root usually retracts. But the gap or weakness in the disc's firm outer ring remains. Any wrong movement can make the pain come back. You can't believe it could be worse, but the next time, it often is. In fact, each episode usually gets a little more severe. So you have a real, super reason to keep that goo in place.

EXERCISES TO PREVENT RECURRENT DISC ATTACKS

One of the best ways to stabilize your spine is to strengthen your abdominal muscles. Slim as those muscles are, they have tremendous leverage. The rib cage above and the pelvis below act just like the handles on a monkey wrench to let your abdominal muscles control movement of the lower spine.

A special exercise lets you strengthen those muscles without the possibility of painful or injurious back movement.

Solution 2

1. Lie on your bed. Bend your knees and plant your feet flat on the bed surface. Place the heel of each hand on the corresponding knee (Figure 8).

2. Lift your head off the bed. Push your right hand hard against your right knee for 10 seconds. While still keeping your head raised, push your left hand against your left knee for 10 seconds.

3. Let your head fall back and rest for 10 seconds.

4. Repeat five times.

You should do this at least twice a day, when you go to bed and when you wake up. One virtue of this exercise is that you don't have to build up the number of repetitions. As you get stronger, the intensity of each contraction will increase, automatically suiting the effort to your capacity.

When you have a ruptured or bulging disc, you want to shift weight from the front part of your vertebrae (where the discs are) to the back. This is exactly the reverse

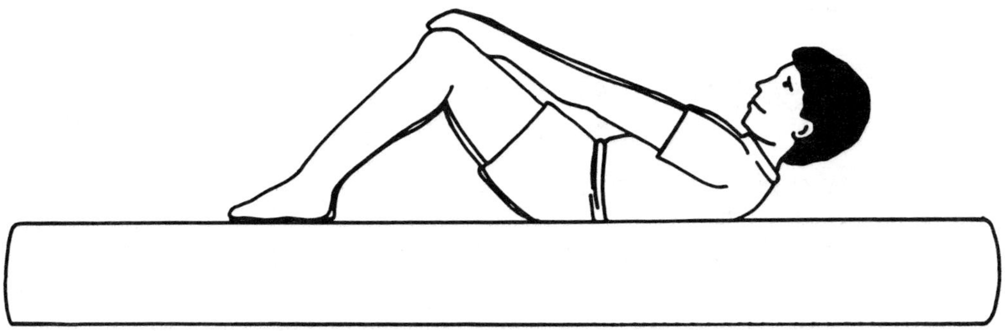

Figure 8

of what you may have learned for avoiding <u>ordinary</u> backstrain.

The next set of exercises will help you to establish the correct posture for avoiding back strain caused by a ruptured or bulging disc.

<u>Solution 3</u>

1. <u>Stretching exercises play a big part in establishing new posture</u>. Muscles only stretch well when they are warm, so you should exercise by walking, riding a

stationary bicycle, or the like before each session.

2. Before your pelvis can tilt forward to shift weight to the back part of your lumbar vertebrae, you need to stretch the muscles at the back of your thighs and those of your calves.
3. Fold a towel until it is eight or ten layers thick.
4. Lie on the floor with your left hip close to a door jamb, with the folded towel underneath your lower back.
5. Stretch your left leg up along the door jamb.
6. Press your knee to straighten your leg totally.
7. Relax and repeat three times.
8. Shift to the other side of the door and repeat the procedure with your right leg.
9. Next, stand facing the wall at arm's length.
10. Put both hands on the wall.
11. Move your left foot back about 2 feet.
12. Keeping your left knee straight, bend your right knee so that your weight presses your left foot up toward your shin, stretching your calf muscles.
13. Repeat three times.

14. Follow the same procedure with your right foot back.

IMPROVED BODY MECHANICS

At the same time, you can do the following exercises to learn new patterns of body movement:

Solution 4

1. Kneel on all fours.
2. Place a rolling pin lengthwise along your lower spine.
3. Without making the rolling pin move, simultaneously lift your right arm and your left leg level with your body.
4. Return to starting position. Simultaneously lift your left arm and right leg. Return to start, and repeat three times.
5. Next, learn to lift and stoop by bending your legs instead of your back using a broomstick or mop handle.
6. Hold one end at the back of your neck with your right hand.
7. Hold the other end against the base of your spine with your left hand.
8. Do a deep knee bend without letting your lower back get any closer to the stick than it is when you are upright. Repeat three

times (and try to use exactly the same technique whenever you stoop or lift).

These exercises help a lot. You should do them twice daily and continue them until the patterns of movement have been thoroughly ingrained.

THE DISC RETRACTING DANGLE

A further helpful procedure was first discovered by an athlete who found that he could relieve his back pain by hanging for long periods from a high gymnastic bar. That's too tough for most people, so I've developed a method that gives a similar effect without needing any strength.

Solution 5

1. Measure the circumference of your chest (below the breasts if you're a woman).
2. Obtain a "pelvic traction belt" to fit your chest measurement[1], a camp-style (canvas

[1]A "pelvic traction belt" is made for a different type of treatment, where pull on your spine comes from weights on pulleys at the foot of the bed. At this writing, I can't find anyone who makes a similar device for pulling upward on the chest. The "pelvic traction belts" available at hospital supply stores or from Scott Specialties, Inc., P.O. Box 129, Belleville, Kansas 66935, (913) 527-5480, can be made to fit

stretched on a frame) cot, and two screw hooks substantially larger than the cot frame. (The "belt" is a padded wide band with broad Velcro® attaching surfaces, allowing considerable adjustment for your body contours including your breasts if you're a woman.)

3. Lean the cot at a 45° angle and against a wall and support its top end (with the legs collapsed) in that position with the screw hooks.

4. If you're a large-breasted woman or a substantially overweight man, wearing a support garment underneath the belt may make it more comfortable and effective.

5. Secure the straps from the traction belt to the screw hooks, adjusting their length so that the belt falls at chest level while you lie on the cot, on tiptoe on the floor.

6. Let all the air out of your lungs and wrap the belt snugly around your chest.

7. Bend your knees, so that the weight of your lower quarters exerts pull on the lower spine.

---

the chest comfortably, however. Attach padding if necessary, especially in the upper sizes, which taper in the wrong direction.

8. Remain in this position (Figure 9) for at least half an hour. You can pull up on the traction straps or on the head of the cot to relieve the pressure at intervals.

If pain and muscle spasm keep this approach from doing the trick, you can increase its action in two ways:

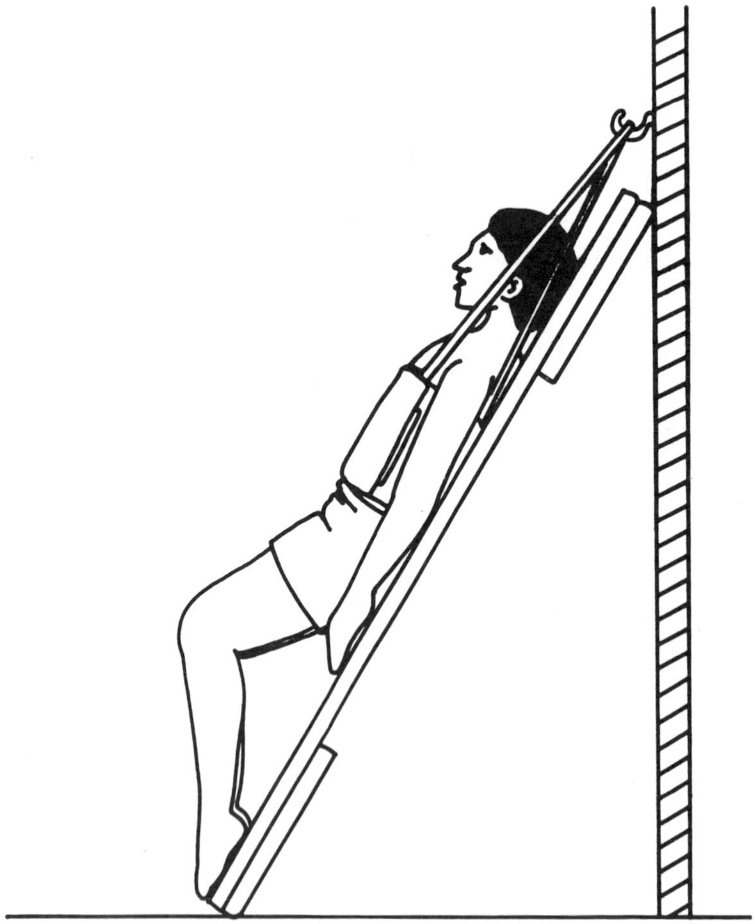

Figure 9

Solution 6:

1. To intensify the disc-retracting dangle, first try to relax your back muscles. You'll find it very difficult to loosen up when you're in pain, but by following the technique described in Solution 7 of Section Two (relaxing your other muscles in rotation until you finally get to your back), you can accomplish more than you expect.

2. If you have muscle relaxants on hand from previous attacks, take full doses half an hour before dangling.

3. Otherwise, take aspirin in the amounts I suggested in Solution 3, Section Three.

4. Mild increase in disc suction can be obtained just by lying on a very slippery cloth. Less friction between your back and the cot means more downward push.

5. If you both need and can stand maximum effect, you can brace the cot in a more erect position by moving the screw eyes.

A "GOO REPLACEMENT" TECHNIQUE

Whenever you have active pain from a disc problem, try adding this technique, which increases negative pressure in the disc and draws the errant goo back into place.

Solution 7

1. While dangling on your cot, very gently roll your hips from side to side. Since ideally you are relaxing at the same time, it helps to have someone else take care of the movements. Just bend your knees to a 30° angle and let your helper hold them together and move them first to the left, then to the right (Figure 10).

2. For the first few days, roll only 10° to 15°.

3. Increase gradually, perhaps another 5° every three days, to a maximum of 45° each way.

4. If you have no helper, make these movements yourself. Steady the upper part of your body with your hands on the screw hooks, so that all the turning movement must take place in the spine.

5. Repeat ten times.

It astonished me to see a "For Sale" sign on Jim G.'s farm. Just one year before, when he hit 40, Jim had told me how much he loved it.

But back trouble had driven him into a corner. After five spells with a ruptured disc, he didn't dare do half the jobs which running the place entailed. And his father had gone through four back operations without getting relief. Even though he knew that surgery has advanced a

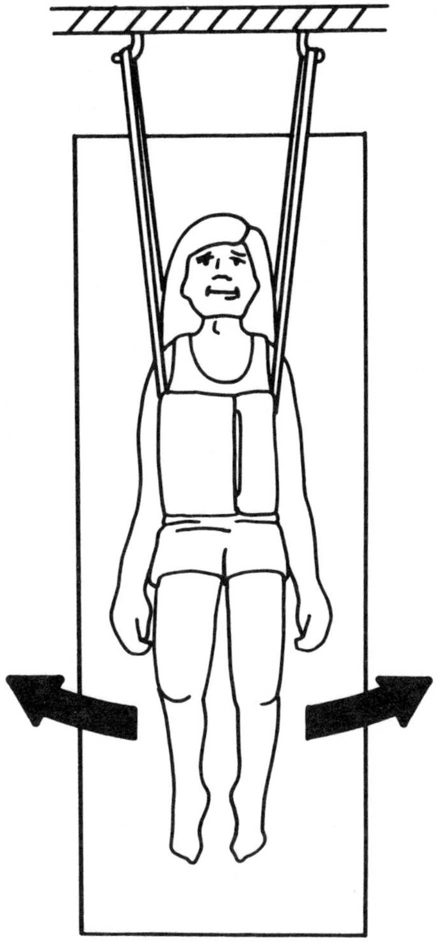

Figure 10

lot since then, Jim couldn't bring himself to climb on the table.

It just happened that Jim came to my office about then for a mild illness. We got to talking about his back, and I suggested the dangle, with hip-rolling as an adjunct. Jim modified the plan to avoid need for a cot: he used the slippery grain-loading chute instead. His wife helped him with the hip-rolling, while he concentrated on staying relaxed.

After a couple of weeks, he took down the "For Sale" sign. That was eight years ago, and he's still running the farm. He still dangles almost every day. I keep reminding him to continue with this remedy, because people tend to slack off once they stop hurting. But he tells me not to bother—that his wife finds him so much easier to live with when he's free of back pain that she isn't likely to let him forget.

SECTION SIX'S KEY POINTS

A ruptured or bulging disc can press on nerves in your back, making pain shoot all the way down to your ankle.

Bed rest in the jackknife position with full doses of aspirin helps you to get over the attack. Special exercises, different from those used for ordinary backstrain, help you to avoid recurrences.

The disc-retracting dangle also helps. Use it both to get over the attack and to keep the pain from coming back. Muscle relaxation, either through the technique described in Solution 7 of Section Two or through whatever muscle relaxants you might have on hand, makes this more effective. So does the hip-rolling technique described in Solution 6.

SECTION SEVEN

HOW TO *PREVENT* BACK PROBLEMS

If you get ordinary backaches often, you'll spend a lot less time and effort in the long run by trying to prevent them rather than waiting until you need to treat them. The techniques that prevent muscular backaches also make back strains and sprains less likely. However, they do not prevent disc problems. If you have a ruptured or bulging disc, follow Section Six's posture control (Solution 2) and body mechanics (Solution 3) methods rather than those in this section.

IMPROVED POSTURE

The more your lower back curves, the harder its muscles have to work, and the more prone it is to strains. When your spine is almost straight, vertebrae sit on top of each other like a stack of blocks. It takes very little muscular effort to keep them there, and both work-weary backaches and actual injuries are much less likely. Here's one very effective method of posture correction:

Solution 1

1. With your heels about 8 inches from a smooth wall, lean back against that surface.

2. Put your hand into the gap between the wall and your lower back to see how much space is there.

3. Now try to reduce that space by two maneuvers:

   - Lift the top of the back of your head as far as possible toward the ceiling.

   - At the same time, tilt your hips forward (Figure 11).

4. When you have narrowed the gap between your lower back and the wall as much as possible, rock forward away from the wall and try to keep your head and back in the same position.

5. Repeat this many times a day until the straight spine posture becomes ingrained. This might be every 5 or 10 minutes the first day, less and less often as time goes on.

6. You will probably need about a month to establish the new posture thoroughly—longer if weak muscles need to be strengthened before you can improve posture to the maximum.

I was at Johns Hopkins Medical School when I learned about these exercises. I backed against a wall and found I could put my whole fist in the gap behind my lumbar spine. I did exactly what I've suggested you should

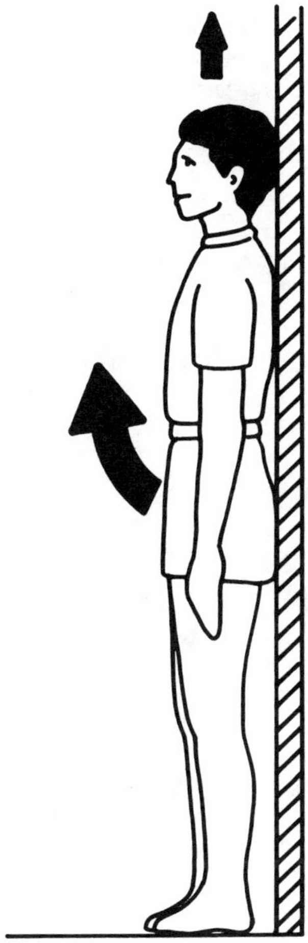

Figure 11

do—walked away from the wall twenty times a day at first. In six weeks, I could hardly get one finger into the gap, and my back has stayed straight without further effort ever since.

I'm sure this has saved me a lot of discomfort and quite possibly some injuries (because a straight back is more stable as well as stronger). It can do the same for you, if you're willing to spend a few hours now to avoid possible weeks of pain later.

STRENGTHENING ABDOMINAL MUSCLES

You'll also find that building up the strength of your abdominal muscles helps to straighten and support your back. Although these are lighter than your back muscles, they have the rib cage above and the pelvis below as levers.

When polio raged, victims whose abdominal muscles were paralyzed got much more curvature of the spine than did those whose back muscles were hit. This shows just how much back support your abdominal muscles give.

Plain old flab can make your back hurt two ways: by contributing to extra curvature and by leaving your spine without muscular support. That's what happened to Mike B, for instance. Mike almost lost his farm when he had a long siege with hepatitis. He got over the attack on time for spring planting, but constant back pain made it almost impossible to get the crops in.

Mike's back hurt when he rode the tractor. It hurt when he lifted bags of seed. After a while, it hurt even when he stopped for a rest or a snack. But he didn't have either a back injury or residuals from his liver infection. He just had weak muscles from months of enforced rest.

Mike had thought that the work itself would soon get his muscles in shape. He couldn't believe that exercises would do much for him. But I convinced him to give this method a try:

<u>Solution 2</u>

1. Start by just lying on your back and raising your head ten times. Do this four times a day for three days. Then go on to the next step.

2. Lie on the floor with your knees bent to a 45° angle and your feet hooked under a heavy piece of furniture. Lock your hands behind your head.

3. Draw your body into a sitting position. Lower your upper body slowly back down onto the floor. This is called a straight situp. Repeat five times.

4. From the same starting position, touch your right elbow to your left knee. Lower your body back down to the floor. Touch your left elbow to your right knee. This is called a turning situp. Repeat five times.

5. On the next day, perform straight and turning situps six times instead of five. Increase by one repetition a day until you reach thirty.

6. If at any time you find your abdominal muscles sore, remain at the same repetition level for three days.

7. Continue to do thirty repetitions of each exercise daily.

After a few weeks, Mike came back to report on his progress. Within a week of starting the exercises, his backaches had almost disappeared. He had gotten all the crops planted and felt sure he could save the farm.

CORRECTING SHORT LEG IMBALANCE

If your back gets tired and hurts whenever you stand up for long, weak muscles may be the problem. But there's also a considerable chance that one leg (usually the left) is shorter than the other. This tilts the base on which your spine rests, so that it needs to curve to keep your weight in balance.

Even half an inch difference in leg length makes enough strain that even good strong muscles begin to ache. While any of the ways of moving out lactic acid that I've told you about will give relief, it's certainly better to prevent this pain altogether. So if you often get backaches from standing, you should check yourself for this condition. Just lie straight on your back. Get someone to measure each leg from the rim of your pelvis to the bottom edge of your outer ankle bone with a tape measure.

If you find a half inch or more difference, follow this technique:

<u>Solution 3</u>

1. Stand with the heel of your shorter leg on a stack of magazines.
2. Add to the stack until you find the thickness which puts both sides of your pelvic rim at the same level (and also makes you most comfortable).
3. Get a shoemaker to put a wedge on the heel of the appropriate shoe. The wedge should be as thick as your magazine stack at the back, and should taper ⅛ inch at the front so that the edge of the heel won't catch as you walk.

LESS WEIGHT, LESS BACK STRAIN

Even if your spine is perfectly straight, its joints may be overburdened. When your weight gets above a certain point, it mashes out the natural lubricant your body puts between the surfaces of your weight-bearing joints. This is like loading up a car until the fenders scrape the wheels: it leads to disproportionate wear and tear.

"But I've tried to hold my weight down," you might say. "It just doesn't work."

You've probably had a hard time losing or keeping weight off. But don't let past failure discourage you. Weight control to get rid of pain or disease involves completely different psychology than weight control for cosmetic reasons or general disease prevention. You will get behind the effort, with no foot dragging. You can use any reduction program you want, from Scarsdale to Ultraslim; they'll all work better when you're keeping pain at bay.

Even if your weight falls inside the "normal" range, you'll often find that backaches disappear or become much milder with loss of a few pounds. Unless you're already really underweight, taking off 5 or 10 pounds often does wonders for your aching back.

UNBURDENING YOUR BACK WITH PROPER LIFTING

Better lifting methods certainly help you to avoid both

muscular backaches and back injuries, including a ruptured disc.

Solution 4

1. Always use your leg muscles rather than your back muscles to lift or push.

2. Keep your back as straight as possible, neither bending nor arching it.

3. Check your footing before starting to lift or push. Use sand, gravel, friction pads, or special footwear to improve traction if necessary.

4. Never lift heavy objects unless you can plant your feet very close to them. For example, don't lift heavy objects out of a car trunk.

5. Use ropes with pulleys, crowbars, or improvised ramps so that you can lift or pull from a more balanced position.

6. Set up simple hoists wherever you frequently need to lift heavy objects.

One of my patients keeps a pallet in the trunk of her car. She has pulleys which attach to it in her garage. Instead of leaning forward in a clumsy position to lift out her groceries, she hooks up the ropes and pulls.

She set up this device <u>after</u> she strained her back and found she couldn't lift any longer. Perhaps you should do it before injury forces you to do so.

At age 45, Joe K. had been working in a warehouse for twenty years. During that time, he lifted literally tons of material, yet he never had a moment's pain in his back. Joe gives credit to three things:

1. Great instruction. His plant safety officer not only tells them, he also shows them exactly how to lift with their legs instead of their back, and which shoe soles will keep their feet firmly planted while they lift.

2. Constant attention to good footing and lifting posture. Joe always has his feet planted, and planted right against the object he's lifting. He never leans over and lifts.

3. Use of equipment. Joe never heaves anything up by hand when a forklift or hoist will do the job.

Joe used to worry about what he would do when he got too old to heave around those boxes. He doesn't have to worry any more. With worker's compensation claims kicking the company's costs sky high, the boss decided he needed a foreman who would push safety above even production.

So Joe's safety record won him a promotion to foreman, where he knows he's good for another twenty years.

USING A CHAIR WITH PROPER SUPPORT

Sometimes you get a "muscular backache" even when you've been continuously seated. This happens when your chair puts muscles under strain instead of relaxing them.

<u>What you feel</u>:

Dull, steady back pain whenever you sit in a certain chair.

<u>Cause</u>:

Improper support. Certain chairs almost force you into a slumped posture which ultimately causes backache.

<u>Solution 5</u>

1. You'll usually find that a comfortable chair has to either keep you upright, so that your vertebrae remain stacked one on top of the other, or support the entire length of your spine.
2. Try to use chairs which reach at least to your shoulder blades, so that they can support your whole back.
3. If you need to use a short-backed chair (perhaps an office-supplied chair or

kitchen stool) set the back so that it presses firmly against the top of your pelvis, not against the hollow in your back.

4. If the chair won't adjust in this way, attach firm sponge rubber pads or use cushions.

5. The way you sit makes a difference, too: try to sit tall. If your chair has a high back, press your lower spine (not your shoulder blades) against its support.

I remember overhearing my secretary say that her back was "killing her" while she was sitting at her desk. When I asked her about it, she said that she got backache whenever she sat there for more than an hour at a time.

"Let's try adjusting your chair," I said. "Maybe it's not giving you enough support."

We tried different back pad and seat heights until we found settings which held her back straight instead of pushing on the lower back's hollow. She worked for me ten more years without ever complaining of backache.

SECTION SEVEN'S KEY POINTS

An ounce of prevention is worth a pound of cure.

- You can learn to hold your spine straight,

so that your vertebrae balance on one another like a stack of blocks. Then your muscles hardly have to work at all. Do the "walk away from the wall" exercise until a straighter spine becomes ingrained.

- Support your back with abdominal muscles that you've strengthened with the exercises in Solution 2.

- If one of your legs proves to be shorter than the other, wear appropriate wedges on your heels.

- Losing even a few pounds can make a huge difference. Knowing that your back will really hurt less if you lose weight helps you accomplish that goal.

- Adjusting your chair and "sitting tall" can keep you from getting backaches from prolonged sitting.

SECTION EIGHT

HOW TO TELL IF DOCTORS CAN GIVE FURTHER HELP

As a family physician, I've always played two separate roles. I've done what I could to cure you. Then I've arranged for experts to give further care if needed.

In this final section, I'm going to play that second role for you. In some instances, I'm going to tell you that your doctor can give further help with a prescription-only medicine. In others, I'm going to tell you what further measures a physical therapist or surgeon might use to get rid of problems which home measures haven't cured.

MUSCULAR BACKACHES FROM BODY IMBALANCE

At 24, Jody V. looked the picture of health. A physical therapist who jogged, hiked, and skied to stay in shape all year long, her muscles couldn't have been firmer.

But she still had backaches every single day, and she had figured out the reason for herself. Jody's breasts were very large. With 32-inch hips and a 24-inch waist, she wore a 38 D brassiere.

She had tried all kinds of support garments without

relief, and finally decided on breast reduction surgery. Actually, she had already arranged this before she came to me, but her health insurance company thought that the operation might be "cosmetic" and therefore not covered by her policy. They sent her to me for evaluation.

When I certified her medical (not cosmetic) need, the insurance company agreed to pay, and Jody had her operation. She hasn't had a backache since.

I talked to her surgeon later. He performs over twice as many operations to reduce breast size as to increase it. And virtually all these patients come because of back pain, not appearance.

ONE VERY SHORT LEG

We talked before about how a short leg could throw you out of balance enough to cause backaches. What if an injury leaves you with a leg too short for an ordinary heel wedge? Maybe you can control the problem with special shoes. Some orthopedic appliance dealers can get shoes constructed with internal pads to correct up to 2 inches of shortness.

An alternative to consider, especially if the injury occurs while one is still growing, is to shorten the longer leg to match. During adolescence surgeons can do this with very little pain or disability by stapling across a growth plate on the longer leg. If timed when just enough growth would normally remain, this gets the two limbs in balance and corrects a problem which would otherwise plague you the rest of your life. When you've stopped growing, it's a tougher operation with a longer convalescence, but still may be worth it.

BACKACHES FROM TENSION

If you go to a doctor for backache caused by nervous tension, chances are the doctor will prescribe a tranquilizer or muscle relaxant. That's one route to relief, but usually a self-perpetuating one.

Constant nervous tension generally amounts to a scream for help. Your body is trying to tell you something. "Get a new job" or "Don't smolder—get the things that peeve you on the table" or "You're living above your means—get your finances rearranged." If you know what's bugging you, but can't find the answer, a specific type of counselor might help: You'll find vocational, family, and financial experts in community agencies or private practice (see the Yellow Pages).

Take Jerry P.'s case, for example. I treated Jerry

for tension-related back pain for several weeks before learning what was bugging him. When I felt that I knew him well enough to "get personal," we finally had a frank, open talk. It turned out that he had so many bills he didn't know what to do. Just after he and his wife bought a car and new furniture, she lost her job and then became pregnant. All he could think of was bills, bills, bills.

I arranged for Jerry to see a budget counsellor at the Family Counseling Bureau. They worked out a debt consolidation plan which kept the payments at a level Jerry could live with and got his household on a sound financial basis.

A few months later, Jerry reported that he hadn't had any more trouble with his back. His wife had found part-time work, and they were ahead of schedule on getting out of debt. And he was concentrating so much better at work that he actually got a promotion.

It's always better to get to the root of things than to just ease current complaints. That holds for emotional as well as physical upsets. Sometimes your pride puts up a big barrier (especially if your personal relationships or your ability to manage your money is involved). But it's better to get help than to struggle endlessly on and on.

BACK STRAIN

If you're injured at work, you almost need to see a doctor. You need papers to get time off from work and a record in case you don't get well promptly. It's a good idea to follow up until you're entirely well; "minor" injuries sometimes turn out to be worse than they seem.

If you need stronger pain medicines or muscle relaxants than you can buy without a prescription, you'll benefit from a doctor's care. You can usually get what you need from a family doctor, walk-in clinic, or emergency room without going to the extra expense of seeing a specialist.

If you have one or more spots on your injured back which prove very tender, a doctor can give you a lot of relief by injecting local anesthetic solution into those spots. Numbing those "trigger points" seems to break a vicious pain-spasm-pain circle. The anesthetic itself only lasts for an hour or so, but breaking the pain-spasm-more pain circle gives relief that often lasts for days from this simple, safe procedure.

ARTHRITIS

If home measures don't control arthritis of your spine, you can expect these forms of help from your physician:

- Inflammation-fighting medicines. Other agents stronger than aspirin or ibuprofen have come into use in recent years. You need a prescription to take one of these, so you'll need to see your doctor.

- Deep heat machines like ultrasound (using the same principle as your microwave oven) can heat tissue deep inside your body.

- Braces or appliances are used sometimes for your comfort and sometimes to keep your back in the right position in case some joints freeze.

- If all else fails, specialists can use a gadget on the end of a needle to desensitize the nerves to your facet joints. They can't kill those nerves altogether or you would always feel numb. But they can cut the pain by 80% or so without any cutting or disability whatever.

OSTEOPOROSIS

Unless she takes replacement hormones, a woman whose ovaries are removed at an early age almost inevitably gets osteoporosis within a few years. Men also get this disorder, especially if body build, skin tone, past diet, and lack of exercise puts them in a high-risk group. But the loss of hormonal support that makes a postmenopausal woman's bones thin out can be remedied. If you're a woman who has passed the menopause, hormone replacement might well save you from bowed back, fractured wrists or hips, and other osteoporotic problems.

If you are in the highest-risk group, or have actual evidence of osteoporosis (including past fracture of a wrist or hip), you will definitely benefit from hormones. Otherwise, you might find yourself on the fence about them. Perhaps you will get enough hot flashes and other menopausal complaints to want relief, but hang back for fear of hormone-spurred breast or uterine cancer.

I can understand why increasing your risk of cancer

even slightly through hormone therapy would make you uneasy. But lack of hormones can cause serious difficulties, too. Hip fractures and heart attacks, for example, definitely happen more often when missing hormones aren't replaced. Statistics prove that hormone replacement has a positive, not a negative, effect on life expectancy. Altogether you gain more than you lose if you take estrogen and progesterone when you need relief from even mild menopause-related complaints.

Note that I said estrogen and progesterone. These two hormones which your ovaries normally supply throughout your reproductive years work together to fight osteoporosis and heart disease. But many doctors prescribe estrogen alone unless you specifically ask for the progesterone (or mention osteoporosis), since that's the "old standby" for hot flashes. If you're going to take estrogen anyway, taking the combination of both major female sex hormones involves no extra side effects or expense and gives much better protection against weakened bone structure.

Whether you're a man or a woman, there's one other possible bone-firming medicine available. That's fluorine, the same stuff you use (whether you want to or not, because it is added to your water supply) to harden the enamel on your teeth. This method is a bit tricky, because too much fluorine causes a painful joint condition and other side effects. The dose has to be adjusted for your size, your salt consumption, other fluorine or fluoride intake (present and past), and any medicines you are taking. You may even need to go to a teaching or research center to get this treatment. But if you have substantial risk (or present evidence) of osteoporosis, this method may prove very helpful.

NERVE ROOT PRESSURE

If you have a bulging or ruptured disc, I certainly hope that rest in jackknife position and the disc-refracting dangle do you some good. But I don't always expect these measures to cure you.

Tim J., for instance, used every technique I've described in this book (and several others, too), but he still had back trouble. Tim worked very hard to get his marina going before he reached age 40. That hard work took its toll: he had suffered three severe episodes of back pain from a ruptured disc, with milder spasms almost every week.

Tim had done everything short of surgery to relieve the situation. He got fair results from dangling—better than he had with other measures on previous attacks. But he kept throwing his back out again, causing more misery and lost time until he seriously considered selling out and looking for lighter work.

Tim's favorite uncle had back surgery years ago. He had four operations with no lasting relief. With that kind of background, I could understand why Tim had hung back from even investigating his condition. But I finally persuaded him that doctors can do a lot better job now that they can see beforehand what they're getting into.

When disc surgery first started, nobody could see a ruptured or bulging disc. X rays only showed bone, not either the firm cartilage of the disc's ring or the soft goo that belonged in its center. So surgeons only had vague changes in reflexes and sensation to tell them what was pressing on which nerve.

Then they thought they had found a very helpful technique. By injecting a dye called Lipiodol into the spinal column, they could often see a gap in the dye, like a glass bead in a bottle of milk, where the disc goo protruded. But Lipiodol turned out to be a time bomb.

Years later, it created scar tissue which pressed on nerves just the way a new disc would. Doctors blamed past surgery for the scar tissue before they learned what really caused it and kept using the Lipiodol for years.

I could tell Tim that the situation today is completely different from that his uncle met. No more groping in the dark—computerized axial tomography (CAT) scans and magnetic resonance imaging show up every bit of tissue. No more time bomb oil-soluble dyes—any dyes used dissolve in water, so that your body can carry them promptly away. Much gentler means of removing cartilage are available—sometimes by surgery under a microscope, sometimes even without any surgery at all, by injecting an enzyme which dissolves the goo inside a bulging (not a ruptured) disc.

Actually, Tim's scans showed a bad situation. One of his discs had ruptured, and the protruding goo was pressing on a major lumbar nerve. So he wound up with an operation after all.

"But it wasn't any where near as bad as I expected," he told me a few months later. "The specialist used microsurgery, where he actually worked with a microscope. Guess he got every bit of the bad stuff out of there, because I haven't had a twinge since. And I'm hauling more boats and motors around than ever. The marina's going great guns since I can really take care of things."

Even the world's greatest surgeons still don't win them all. But they do much better than they did even a few years ago. Don't let the bad experiences others have had in past years scare you off. If there's a substantial chance that specialized treatment can help you, at least have the tests you need to tell what's going on. Don't suffer for years when today's experts could heal you, just because yesterday's experts did not have the advantages of recent advances.

When I first started in practice, I sent patients to a surgeon only if their pain kept them in bed more than six weeks a year for several years. In those early days of disc surgery, the specialists were all anxious to show what they could do, which made them downright knife happy. And what they could do was grope in the dark—X rays showed only bone shadows, not the disc itself, and they really couldn't see what they were doing when they scraped away at the bottom of a deep incision.

Doctors have made a lot of progress since then, both in nonsurgical and in surgical approaches. If home measures don't do the trick for you, why not see what health professionals can do for you?

SECTION EIGHT'S KEY POINTS

Although you're reading this report mainly to find things you can do for yourself, you may also benefit from knowing what further measures are available.

If large breasts, a short leg, or other forms of body imbalance cause your backaches, special garments or surgical measures might solve your problem. You might also want to see a physical therapist.

Backaches from nervous tension may disappear for good if you resolve the problems that are bothering you. Marriage, vocational, financial, and other types of counselors may put you on track.

Back strain may call for prescription-strength pain medicines or muscle relaxants. "Trigger point" injections often give great relief.

Doctors can fight spinal arthritis with prescription-only inflammation fighters, tissue-heating machines, braces, or pain nerve-desensitizing procedures.

Prescription-only hormones and fluorides help rebuild the thinned bones of osteoporosis.

Ruptured or bulging discs show up clearly on modern-day scans. Goo-dissolving injections might do wonders. And if worst comes to worst, it's nice to know that today's surgeons get much better results than do those of the last generation did.

INDEX

A

B

F

G

H

I

J

L

M

N

O

P

R

S